Bruce + Cyndie
Maryanoff

ORD AND CD IN CHEMISTRY AND BIOCHEMISTRY

An Introduction

ORD AND CD IN CHEMISTRY AND BIOCHEMISTRY

An Introduction

PIERRE CRABBÉ

Syntex, S. A.
Universidad Nacional Autonoma de Mexico
and
Universidad Iberoamericana
Mexico, D. F., Mexico

Academic Press   New York and London   1972

ACADEMIC PRESS, INC.
111 Fifth Avenue, New York, New York 10003

United Kingdom Edition published by
ACADEMIC PRESS, INC. (LONDON) LTD.
24/28 Oval Road, London NW1 7DD

LIBRARY OF CONGRESS CATALOG CARD NUMBER: 79-189163

PRINTED IN THE UNITED STATES OF AMERICA

In memory of my brother Paul

CONTENTS

PREFACE

The purpose of this monograph is to provide an elementary introduction and the minimum theoretical background necessary for the useful application of optical rotatory dispersion (ORD) and circular dichroism (CD) to common chemical problems. Its presentation and content should give a sufficient body of information to familiarize unacquainted students in chemistry and biochemistry with these techniques.

In addition to the infrared (IR) and ultraviolet (UV) techniques, one can now dispose of modern tools such as nuclear magnetic resonance (NMR) spectroscopy, gas-liquid chromatography (GLC), and mass spectrometry (MS). Combined with X-ray crystallography, these methods make that the scientists have available a very powerful and sophisticated armamentarium to solve structural and stereochemical problems. Nevertheless, ORD and CD, the only methods to study chiral molecules by analysis of their Cotton effects, provide valuable information with small amounts of material in a relatively short period of time. Compared to the wealth of information one can get from an NMR or MS, for example, the ORD or CD data may appear restricted or limited, but the acuteness and precision of the stereochemical information they provide have probably no equivalent in chemistry. In fact, the chiroptical methods have witnessed an astounding development, and they are increasingly finding a place as routine and valuable tools in chemistry and biochemistry, from the smallest molecules to various kinds of polycyclic natural products, ligands, biopolymers, and synthetic high polymers.

After the mention of some historical aspects and a brief review of elementary principles of stereochemistry, a short section deals with the phenomena of optical activity and with definitions and units commonly used in ORD and CD. Pertinent references related to theoretical considerations and instruments are mentioned.

So far, the most significant applications of the chiroptical techniques are concerned with organic molecules, thus emphasis will be put on the Cotton effects exhibited by functional groups commonly encountered in organic chemistry. The various octant, quadrant, and sector rules will be mentioned, the most important ones being illustrated with examples. The influence of the nature of the solvent and the effect of temperature on ORD

and CD curves are important factors dealt with separately. The optical properties of polymers, organometallic, and inorganic derivatives are briefly reviewed. A short section reports some aspects of the rapidly developing magnetic optical rotatory dispersion (MORD) and magnetic circular dichroism
(MCD). The Appendix gives the highlights of some salient papers published
lately. Some problems have also been included.

To conclude, a table, which also serves as an index, reports the wavelength range of the Cotton effects of most chromophoric groupings with
relevant references.

This monograph is a slight modification of some notes for students
entitled "An Introduction to the Chiroptical Methods in Chemistry," edited
in Mexico, which has been brought up-to-date with recent references.

I wish to thank several of my students from the University of Mexico
for preparing new compounds for ORD and CD study. Moreover, I express
my gratitude to Drs. E. Bunnenberg, A. Burgstahler, C. Djerassi, Ch. Engel,
A. Moscowitz, K. Nakanishi, H. Ripperger, A. I. Scott, and G. Snatzke for
communicating results and observations prior to publication. Thanks are also
due to Mr. H. Carpio for drawing the figures and formulas. Finally, I should
like to express my special thanks to Miss Xochitl Chavez for her cooperation
in the preparation of this monograph and for typing the entire manuscript.

Pierre Crabbé

I. BASIC PRINCIPLES, DEFINITIONS, AND UNITS

I-1. Historical aspects.

Albeit the fundamental principles of the chiroptical phenomena were discovered more than 150 years ago, it is only during the last fifteen years that ORD and the closely related CD have become widespread physico-chemical tools in chemistry in general and organic chemistry in particular. Table I-1 reports some important historical events related to the development of chiroptical methods (see also ref. 12-15).

Table I-1 of Principal Historical Developments

Date	Authors	Concept	Ref.
1808	Malus	Polarization of light	1
1811	Arago	Changes of optical activity with wavelength (quartz)	2
1813-17	Biot	Optical activity of some organic substances	3
1846	Faraday	Magnetic optical activity	4
1847	Haedinger	Discovery of circular dichroism	5
1896	Cotton	Circular dichroism in solution	6
1933-35	Mitchell, Lowry	First books on the Cotton effect	7
1955	Djerassi	First paper of ORD and CD series by Wayne and Stanford school	8
1955	Rudolph	First commercial ORD instrument	9
1960	Grosjean, Legrand	Application of Pockels effect to CD instrument. First commercial dichrograph	10
1969-71	Mazur, Yogev et al.	First studies in linear dichroism	11

1

I-2. Structure, configuration, conformation.

        To describe fully an organic compound,
one has to define both its structure and stereochemistry (16). First one will specify the
aliphatic, alicyclic, or aromatic system under
investigation, as well as the nature and position of the various functional groups. In order to define the relative or absolute stereochemistry, one has to establish the configuration (α or β, cis or trans, syn or anti, etc.)
of the substituents on the carbon skeleton and
at the ring junctions, and/or on a side chain.
In addition, one has to establish which is the
conformation (chair, boat, twist, etc.) of the
rings. In the case of D-(+)-camphor, the
structure will be defined when one has specified
the alicyclic system, the nature and position of
the various functional groups (carbonyl and
alkyl substituents); i.e., the structure of D-
(+)-camphor is represented by formula (1a).
Then one will specify the configuration of the
methyl at position 1 and the gem-dimethyl
bridge (1b), as well as the boat conformation of
the cyclohexanone ring. Hence, formula (1c)
gives both the structure and stereochemistry of
this cyclic ketone. As will be seen, ORD and
CD can provide valuable structural information.
Nevertheless, it is in stereochemistry that the
optical methods have shown their power (12-15).

1a   1b   1c   2

I-3. Optical rotatory dispersion — Cotton ef-
      fect.

        Compounds capable of rotating the plane
of polarization of light are said to show optical rotatory power and to be optically active.
Such substances may be divided into two main
classes. First, the class in which the optical

rotation is observed in the crystal only, e.g. sodium chlorate, quartz, etc. Second, the group of substances wherein optical activity may be exhibited by the solid, liquid, or gas, either in the pure state or as a solution, In the first class, the ability to rotate the plane of polarization is related to the arrangement of the atoms in the crystal, because this structure disappears on melting; the liquid does not exhibit any optical activity. The compounds of the second type are optically active by virtue of the dissymmetry in the molecule itself and the optical activity is retained in all physical states.

To be optically active, a molecule of the second group should be either chiral or devoid of symmetry elements. A molecule is chiral if it can exist in enantiomeric forms, although it may possess an axis of symmetry (e.g. skewed biaryls). A molecule is asymmetric if it is devoid of a center of inversion, a plane of symmetry, and an alternating rotation – reflection axis of symmetry. This is the case of compounds possessing an asymmetric carbon atom, where the four substituents are different groupings, as in the recently synthetized (+)-bromochlorofluoromethane (2) (17), one of the simplest organic molecules capable of optical activity.

It has been known for a long time that the optical rotatory power of an active substance (solid, liquid, or in solution) varies with the wavelength (λ) of the light passing through it. Indeed, any optically active organic compound presents a specific rotation $[\alpha]_\lambda$ which is a function of the rotation of the plane of polarization, the wavelength (λ) of the incident light, the concentration, and the length of the cell.

The molecular rotation $[\Phi]$ is defined in equation [1]:

$$[1] \qquad [\Phi] \;=\; \frac{[\alpha] \;\cdot\; M}{100}$$

in which M is the molecular weight of the optically active compound.

The changes of optical activity with the wavelengths lead to an optical rotatory dispersion curve. This means that an ORD curve is a function of the difference in refractive index of a substance for left-handed and right-handed circularly polarized light with wavelength. For a compound which does not possess a chromophore (i.e., a substance which does not absorb light) in the spectral region being examined, the optical activity progressively decreases in magnitude as the wavelength increases. Above 300 nm, a positive plain (normal or monotonous positive) ORD curve, such as in (R)-(+)-1-bromofluorenol (3a), or a negative plain (monotonous negative) ORD curve, as in the (S)-(-)-enantiomer (3b) (18) is thus obtained, depending upon whether it rises or falls with decreasing wavelengths (Fig. I-1).

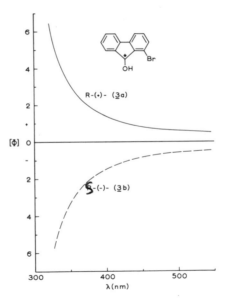

Fig. I-1. Positive plain ORD curve of (R)-(+)-1-bromofluorenol (3a) and negative plain ORD curve of (S)-(-)-bromofluorenol (3b) (18).

Outside the region where optically active absorption bands are observed, Drude (19) proposed the equation [2] which relates the optical activity with the wavelength of the incident light:

$$[2] \qquad [\Phi] = \Sigma \frac{K}{\lambda^2 - \lambda_0^2}$$

where K is a constant depending upon the molecular weight of the optically active compound, λ is the wavelength of the incident light, and λ_0 is the wavelength of the closest absorption maximum. Equation [2] clearly shows that the optical activity enhances with decreasing wavelengths.

If a compound presents one or several optically active absorption bands, its ORD curve will show peaks or troughs in the spectral region in which the chromophores absorb, the ORD curve is then called anomalous: it is a Cotton effect curve.

D-(+)-Camphor (1) contains a carbonyl chromophore absorbing at ca. 292 nm (see UV absorption in Fig. I-2). The keto group is located in a dissymmetric surrounding and thus is optically active. Its ORD curve is characterized by a peak at 312 nm. At lower wavelength (274 nm) there is a trough. The point λ_0 (294 nm) of rotation $[\Phi] = 0°$, where the curve inverts its sign, corresponds roughly to the wavelength of the UV absorption band. The vertical distance between the peak and the trough ("a" in Fig. I-2) is the molecular amplitude, defined as the difference between the molecular rotation at the extremum of longer wavelength $[\Phi]_1$ and the molecular rotation at the extremum of shorter wavelength $[\Phi]_2$, divided by 100, as shown in equation [3]:

$$[3] \qquad a = \frac{[\Phi]_1 - [\Phi]_2}{100}$$

In D-(+)-camphor (1) the molecular amplitude is a + 64 (EtOH).

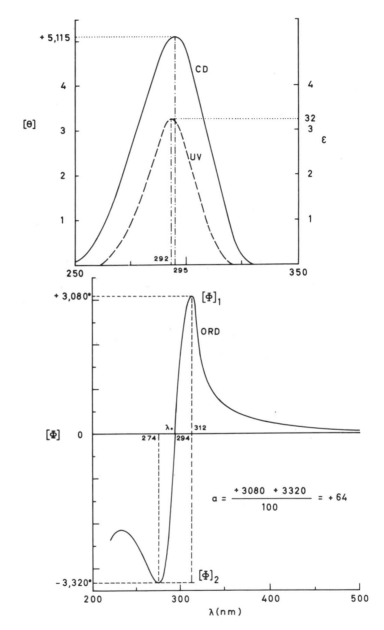

Fig. I-2.   UV and positive Cotton effect ORD and CD curves of D-(+)-camphor (1).

I-4. Circular dichroism - Rotational strength.

Whilst the dispersion effect of an optically active chromophore is attributed to a difference in speed between the circularly polarized beams of light, the circular dichroism effect results from the fact that the right circularly polarized ray is differently absorbed from the left circularly polarized beam of light.
The differential dichroic absorption is defined by equation [4]:

$$[4] \qquad \Delta\varepsilon \;=\; \varepsilon_L \;-\; \varepsilon_R$$

with ε_L and ε_R being the molecular extinction coefficients for the left and right rays.
Another unit commonly used in CD is the molecular ellipticity [Θ] which is related to the differential dichroic absorption $\Delta\varepsilon$ by equation [5]:

$$[5] \qquad [\Theta] \;=\; (\sim 3300) \;.\; \Delta\varepsilon$$

The rotational strength R_k serves to measure the interaction of a chromophore k with its dissymmetric environment. It may also be used as a measure of the asymmetry induced in the electron distribution within the chromophore itself. The rotational strength R_k is equal to the area corresponding to the CD^k band of a given chromophore and is related to the induced electric and magnetic dipole moments by equation [6]:

$$[6] \qquad R_k \;=\; \mu_e^k \;.\; \mu_m^k$$

where μ_e^k and μ_m^k have the dimensions of electric and magnetic dipole moments, respectively.
Fig. I-2 clearly indicates that both ORD and CD curves of D-(+)-camphor (1) display a positive Cotton effect in the region of the UV absorption band. Thus, the sign of the Cotton effect is the same by both methods.

7

Some functions [e.g. a conjugated ketone such as in the steroid (4)] exhibit multiple Cotton effect curves. In this type of ORD curve two or more peaks and troughs are observed. The corresponding multiple Cotton effect CD curve shows various positive and/or negative maxima.

I-5. Comparison between ORD and CD curves.

The information that the chiroptical techniques provide about a particular compound or chromophore is interchangeable, and the relative merits of the two methods are often dependent on the type of instrument being used. The major differences between the information provided by the ORD and CD techniques are of two types. First, an optically active compound devoid of absorption band in the wavelength range under examination will not exhibit any CD effect. However, in spite of the lack of Cotton effect, such a compound will present a plain positive or negative ORD curve, since the rotational contribution of more distant absorption bands gives rise to a background or skeleton effect (reminiscent of the fingerprinting typical of IR spectra). Second, although the sign of the Cotton effect should be the same by CD and ORD, sometimes the shape of the latter curve will be substantially affected by the skeleton effect. This is particularly true in the case of the ORD curves of compounds exhibiting a weak Cotton effect superposed on a strong skeleton effect of opposite sign. As a result, whilst the shape of ORD curves can provide a useful information in structural studies, the precise intensity of weak Cotton effects will be measured more accurately by CD.

Most ORD and CD instruments have been reviewed and discussed in detail (13-15,20).

Since the stereochemistry of steroids and triterpenes is reasonably simple, well established, and the conformation of the polycyclic system rather rigid, it is very fortunate that a considerable part of the work on ORD and CD has been performed in these particular series of natural products. Furthermore, there exists probably no other group of organic compounds for which so much information has been accumulated on chemical and stereochemical features. For this reason, several rules related to optical properties first proposed in the steroid and triterpene fields have turned out later to be of general applicability to all classes of optically active compounds (12).

Figure I-3 reproduces the ORD and CD curves of the 16-hydroxymethyl-isoprogesterone (4), for which a structure published earlier was questionable (21).

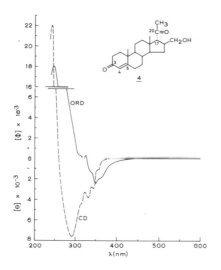

Fig. I-3. ORD and CD curves of 16-hydroxy-methyl-isoprogesterone (4).

Fig. I-3 shows that the CD curve of (4) exhibits at least three different Cotton effects. First, the n-π* and π-π* transitions of the Δ^4-3-keto-chromophore at ca. 350 and 250 nm, respectively. Moreover, the progesterone analogue (4) also presents a Cotton effect in the 300 nm region, typical of the optically active n-π*

9

transition of a saturated ketone, thus excluding
the hemiketal structure proposed earlier. Besides, illustrating an application of CD for the
resolution of a structural problem, Figure I-3
also provides some stereochemical information
about the substituent at C-17. The fact that
the Cotton effect at ca. 300 nm is negative indicates that the configuration of the acetyl side
chain at C-17 is α. Indeed, the octant rule,
which allows one to assign the stereochemistry
around a carbonyl on the basis of the sign of
the Cotton effect (22) (Sec. II-7), predicts
that a negative Cotton effect will be associated
with the 17α-acetyl configuration. Whilst the
CD curve clearly shows the negative Cotton effect associated with the C-20 carbonyl chromophore, it is also apparent from Fig. I-3 that
the ORD curve only presents a shoulder in this
region, because the negative Cotton effect of
the saturated 20-carbonyl at 300 nm is obliter-
ated by a very intense positive Cotton effect in
the 250 nm region, due to the $\pi-\pi^*$ band of the
α,β-unsaturated keto-chromophore. Hence, in the
case of a molecule such as (4) which presents
various absorption bands in a narrow wavelength
range, the CD curve will give a better resolution of the various Cotton effects than the corresponding ORD curve. CD thus provides a more
accurate quantitative value for the various optically active transitions (making CD similar to
UV spectra in this respect) (14,15).
    The optical methods are useful tools in
stereochemistry for the determination of relative and/or absolute configuration and for conformational studies. The correct stereochemistry can either be deduced from the examination
of the experimental Cotton effects in the light
of available octant, quadrant, and sector rules,
or by correlation, i.e., comparison of the optical properties with those of a model compound of
known stereochemistry. Evidently, the chiral
character of the optical methods sets them in a
separate class, as against the other available
physical techniques. As illustrated above, leav-

ing aside the chiral nature of ORD and CD, they can be particularly sensitive proofs for exploring molecular structures. Thus, these techniques are often used in collaboration with the other physical tools, since all of them picture a functional group from a different view point.

I-6. Theoretical aspects.

The theoretical treatment of the chiroptical phenomena offers great difficulties, but rapid advances are now being made, which no doubt will give a new impulse to the ORD and CD techniques. Table I-2 provides a summary of the principal theoretical developments.

Table I-2 of Principal Theoretical Developments

Date	Authors	Concept	Ref.
1823	Fresnel	Optical activity as a function of refractive indices	7,23
1860	Pasteur	Principles of dissymmetry	24
1892	Drude	Dispersion of rotation. Charged particle in helical path	19
1926-1927	Kronig, Kramers	Relationship between absorption and dispersion	25
1928	Rosenfeld	Application of quantum theory; $\mu c.\mu m \not= 0$	26
1929-1930	Kuhn	Classical polarizability; coupled oscillators	27
1930	Lowry	Optically active absorption bands	7
1937	Condon, Altar, Eyring	One-electron model; electron in helical path	28
1937	Kirkwood	Polarizability; coupled oscillators; quantum treatment (exciton theory)	29
1956-1957	Moffitt, Kirkwood	Coupled dipoles (peptides)	30
1957-1961	Moscowitz	Dipole velocity (hexahelicene)	31
1959	Labhart, Wagnière	Non-conjugated dissymmetric chromophores (coupling in β,γ-unsaturated ketones)	32

11

Date	Authors	Concept	Ref.
1960	Tinoco, Woody	μm Treatment. Coupled electric and magnetic dipoles	33
1961–1965	Doty, Holzwarth, et al.	Coupled dipoles. Helical conformation	34
1961	Moffitt, Woodward, Moscowitz, Klyne, Djerassi	Perturbed carbonyl chromophore (octant rule)	22
1961	Cookson, MacKenzie	Coupling of chromophores; charge-transfer (carbonyl)	35
1961	Mislow, Moscowitz, Djerassi et al.	Non-conjugated dissymmetric chromophores	36
1962	Moscowitz	Perturbed chromophore (incompletely screened nuclei)	37
1962	Mason	Coupling of chromophores; charge-transfer	38
1962–1964	Cookson, Hudec	Non-conjugated dissymmetric chromophores (β,γ-unsaturated ketones)	39
1962–1966	Mason et al.	Coupled oscillators (biaryls, diphenylallenes)	40
1964	Caldwell, Eyring	One-electron theory (1-methylindan)	41
1964	Moscowitz et al.	Discussion of charge-transfer (carbonyl)	42a
1965	Moscowitz et al.	Perturbed single chromophore (aromatic)	42b
1965	Charney	Skewed cisoid diene	43
1966–1968	Schellman	Symmetry rules	44
1966	Wagniere	Carbonyl (quadrant rule)	45
1966	Pao, Santry	SCFMO; perturbation through bonds (carbonyl, nodal planes)	46
1966	Allinger, Tai	Carbonyl transition	47
1966	Weigang, Höhn	Carbonyl transition	48
1967	Lynden-Bell, Saunders	SCFMO; perturbation through bonds (extended Hückel treatments of carbonyl octant rule)	49
1967	Oosterhoff et al.	Krönig-Kramers transformation (ORD-CD correlation)	50

I. BASIC PRINCIPLES, DEFINITIONS, AND UNITS

Date	Authors	C o n c e p t	Ref.
1968	Urry	Molecular geometry and optical activity	51
1968	Weigang, Höhn	Synthesis of one-electron and coupled oscillator	52
1970	Hoffmann, Gould	Non planar butadiene	53
1970	Linderberg, Michl	Disulfide	54
1970	Wagnière, Hug	Chromophores of symmetry C_2 (helicenes, dienes, enones, diones)	55
1970	Inskeep, Miles, Eyring	Coupled oscillator calculations of molecules of fixed structure	56
1971	Mayers, Urry	Rotational strength of the peptide transitions	57
1971	Chen, Woody	Calculations of optical properties of poly-L-tyrosine	58

The conventional theory of optical activity is built on the phase difference induced in the beam by the inequality of the refractive indices for circularly polarized light. Briefly, a plane polarized beam of light may be decomposed into two circular components of equal amplitude. When entering a medium, the two components will propagate with the same velocity and on emerging will again propagate with the original velocity: their superimposition is equivalent to an unrotated plane polarized wave (59). However, if the refractive index of the medium depends on the sense of rotation of the electric vector of the incident ray, the two components will propagate with different velocities, and will differ in phase, on emerging after passage through a length of material. The superimposition of the emergent circular components gives rise to a plane polarized beam, but the plane of polarization is rotated from its original direction by an angle which is proportional to the phase difference (59).

The molecular part of the theoretical calculation deals with the refractive index. The molecules that constitute the sample are assumed to be perturbed by the electric and magnetic components of the field of the light wave, and the polarization they induce is calculated and related to the refractive index through the Rosenfeld equation (26).

A transition from the ground state to an excited state in the molecule must be both electric dipole and magnetic dipole allowed and the two transition moments must not be perpendicular. Hence, excitations that may be considered to arise by a helical displacement of charge will have non-zero parallel components and molecules that can allow such excitations will be naturally optically active. Such molecules do not possess centres of inversion or planes of symmetry, and molecules that are mirror images will have opposite signs and so will give equal and opposite optical rotations (59).

An important approach to the calculation

14

of the optical activity of molecules, which can
be divided into several essentially independent
groups, is based on the Rosenfeld equation and
shows that the total activity can be considered
as resulting from four major sources (29,60,61).
The first contribution arises if one of the
groups is inherently dissymmetric. In such a
case the optical rotation angle is due to the
interference of the electric and magnetic transition moments within that group. The second
contribution, so-called one-electron terms, results from the dissymmetry of one group induced
by the others, in such a way that the dissymmetric group so produced behaves as an optically active centre. The other two contributions
are the coupled-oscillator terms, in which
there is an interaction between the transition
moments on separate groups, which are helical
for dissymmetric molecules (59-62).

A complete development of the fundamen-
tals of optical activity, starting from basic
electromagnetic and quantum theory, has appeared recently (62).

References

1. ·E.L. Malus, Mém. Soc. d'Arcueil, 2, 143
   (1808).
2. D.F. Arago, Mém. Inst., 12, 93, 115 (1811).
3. J.B. Biot, Ann. Chim. Phys., 4, 90 (1815);
   Mém. Acad. Sci., 2, 41 (1817).
4. M. Faraday, Phil. Mag., 28, 294 (1846); 29,
   153 (1846); Phil. Trans., 3, 1 (1846).
5. W. Haedinger, Ann. Phys., 70, 531 (1847).
6. A. Cotton, Compt. rend., 120, 989, 1044
   (1895); Ann. Chim. Phys., 8, 347 (1896).
7. S. Mitchell, The Cotton effect, G. Bell,
   London (1933); T.M. Lowry, Optical Rotatory
   Power, Longmans Green and Co., London (1935)
   and Dover Publ. Inc., New York (1954).
8. C. Djerassi, E.W. Foltz, and A.E. Lippman,
   J. Amer. Chem. Soc., 77, 4354 (1955).
9. H.C. Rudolph, J. Opt. Soc. Am., 45, 50
   (1955).

10. M. Grosjean and M. Legrand, Compt. rend.,
    251, 2150 (1960).
11. A. Yogev, L. Margulies, D. Amar, and Y.
    Mazur, J. Amer. Chem. Soc., 91, 4558
    (1969); A. Yogev, L. Margulies, and Y.
    Mazur, J. Amer. Chem. Soc., 93, 249 (1971).
12. C. Djerassi, Optical Rotatory Dispersion:
    Applications to Organic Chemistry, McGraw-
    Hill, New York (1960).
13. L. Velluz, M. Legrand, and M. Grosjean,
    Optical Circular Dichroism. Principles,
    Measurements, and Applications, Verlag
    Chemie, Weinheim (1965).
14. P. Crabbé, Optical Rotatory Dispersion and
    Circular Dichroism in Organic Chemistry,
    Holden-Day, San Francisco (1965); Applica-
    tions de la Dispersion Rotatoire Optique
    et du Dichroïsme Circulaire Optique en
    Chimie Organique, Gauthier Villars, Paris
    (1968).
15. G. Snatzke (edit.) Optical Rotatory Disper-
    sion and Circular Dichroism in Organic Chem
    istry, Heyden and Sons Ltd., London (1967).
16. D.H.R. Barton, Science, 169, 539 (1970);
    J.B. Lambert, Scient. Amer., 222, 58 (1970);
    E.L. Eliel, Stereochemistry of Carbon Com-
    pounds, McGraw-Hill, Inc., New York (1962);
    K. Mislow, Introduction to Stereochemistry,
    W.A. Benjamin, Inc., New York (1965).
17. M.K. Hargreaves and B. Modarai, Chem. Comm.,
    16 (1969); J. Chem. Soc., (C), 1013 (1971).
18. A.C. Darby, M.K. Hargreaves, and D.A. Raval,
    Chem. Comm., 1554 (1970).
19. P. Drude, Nachr. Akad. Wiss. Gottingen, 366
    (1892); Lehrbuch der Optik, S. Hirzel
    Verlag, Leipzig (1906).
20. P. Crabbé and A.C. Parker in Physical Meth-
    ods in Chemistry, A. Weissberger and B.W.
    Rossiter (edit.), Chapt. 3, J. Wiley and
    Sons, Inc., New York (1971).
21. P. Crabbé and J. Romo, Bull. Soc. Chim.
    Belg., 72, 208 (1963).
22. W. Moffitt, R.B. Woodward, A. Moscowitz, W.
    Klyne, and C. Djerassi, J. Amer. Chem. Soc.,

83, 4013 (1961).
23. A. Fresnel, Mémoires, No. 28 (1822); No. 30 (1823); Ann. Chim. Phys., 28, 147 (1825).
24. L. Pasteur, Lectures delivered before the Société Chimique de Paris, January 20 and February 3, 1860.
25. R. de L. Kronig, J. Opt. Soc. Am., 12, 547 (1926); H.A. Kramers, Atti. Congr. Int. Fisici, 2, 545 (1927); see also ref. 50.
26. L. Rosenfeld, Z. Phys., 52, 161 (1928).
27. W. Kuhn, Z. Physikal. Chem., B4, 14 (1929); Trans. Faraday Soc., 26, 293 (1930); Stereochemie, K. Freudenberg (edit.), Deuticke, Leipzig (1933).
28. E.U. Condon, W. Altar, and H. Eyring, J. Chem. Phys., 5, 753 (1937).
29. J.G. Kirkwood, J. Chem. Phys., 5, 479 (1937).
30. W. Moffitt, J. Chem. Phys., 25, 467 (1956); W. Moffitt, D.D. Fitts, and J.G. Kirkwood, Proc. Natl. Acad. Sci. U.S., 43, 723 (1953).
31. A. Moscowitz, Ph.D. Thesis, Harvard University (1957); Tetrahedron, 13, 48 (1961); see also ref. 37.
32. H. Labhart and G. Wagnière, Helv. Chim. Acta., 42, 2219 (1959).
33. I. Tinoco, J. Chem. Phys., 33, 1332 (1960); 34, 1067 (1961); I. Tinoco and R.W. Woody, J. Chem. Phys., 32, 461 (1960); R.W. Woody and I. Tinoco, J. Chem. Phys., 46, 2927 (1967).
34. W.B. Gratzer, G. Holzwarth, and P. Doty, Proc. Natl. Acad. Sci. U.S., 47, 1785 (1961); G. Holzwarth, W.B. Gratzer, and P. Doty, J. Amer. Chem. Soc., 84, 3194 (1962); K. Rosenheck and P. Doty, Proc. Natl. Acad. Sci. U.S., 47, 1775 (1961); G. Holzwarth and P. Doty, J. Amer. Chem. Soc., 87, 218 (1965).
35. R.C. Cookson and S. MacKenzie, Proc. Chem. Soc., 423 (1961).
36. K. Mislow, M.A.W. Glass, A. Moscowitz, and C. Djerassi, J. Amer. Chem. Soc., 83, 2771 (1961); 84, 1945 (1962).

37. A. Moscowitz in Advances in Chemical
     Physics, Prigogine (edit.), vol. 4, I, p.
     67, Interscience Publ., New York (1962).
38. S.F. Mason, Mol. Phys., 5, 343 (1962);
     Quart. Rev., 17, 20 (1963).
39. R.C. Cookson and J. Hudec, J. Chem. Soc.,
     429 (1962).
40. S.F. Mason and G.W. Vane, Tetrahedron Let-
     ters, 1593 (1965); J. Chem. Soc. (B), 370
     (1966); S.F. Mason, G.W. Vane, K. Schofield,
     R.J. Wells, and J.S. Whitehurst, J. Chem.
     Soc. (B), 553 (1967).
41. D.J. Caldwell and H. Eyring, Ann. Rev. Phys.
     Chem., 15, 281 (1964); H. Eyring, H.C. Liu,
     and D. Caldwell, Chem. Rev., 68, 525 (1968).
42a. A. Moscowitz, A.E. Hansen, L.S. Forster,
     and K. Rosenheck, Biopolymers, Symp., No. 1,
     75 (1964).
42b. A. Moscowitz, A. Rosenberg, and A.E. Hansen,
     J. Amer. Chem. Soc., 87, 1813 (1965).
43. E. Charney, Tetrahedron, 21, 3127 (1965).
44. J.A. Schellman, J. Chem. Phys., 44, 55
     (1966); Acc. Chem. Res., 1, 144 (1968).
45. G. Wagnière, J. Amer. Chem. Soc., 88, 3937
     (1966).
46. Y.H. Pao and D.P. Santry, J. Amer. Chem.
     Soc., 88, 4157 (1966).
47. J.C. Tai and N.L. Allinger, J. Amer. Chem.
     Soc., 88, 2179 (1966).
48. O.E. Weigang and E.G. Höhn, J. Amer. Chem.
     Soc., 88, 3673 (1966).
49. R.M. Lynden-Bell and V.R. Saunders, J. Chem.
     Soc. (A), 2061 (1967).
50. C.A. Emeis, L.J. Oosterhoff, and G. de
     Vries, Proc. Roy. Soc. A, 297, 54 (1967).
51. D.W. Urry, Ann. Rev. Phys. Chem., 19, 477
     (1968).
52. E.G. Höhn and O.E. Weigang, J. Chem. Phys.,
     48, 1127 (1968).
53. R.R. Gould and R. Hoffmann, J. Amer. Chem.
     Soc., 92, 1813 (1970).
54. J. Linderberg and J. Michl, J. Amer. Chem.
     Soc., 92, 2619 (1970).

55. G. Wagnière and W. Hug, Tetrahedron Letters, 4765 (1970); Helv. Chim. Acta, 54, 633 (1971).
56. W.H. Inskeep, D.W. Miles, and H. Eyring, J. Amer. Chem. Soc., 92, 3866 (1970).
57. D.F. Mayers and D.W. Urry, Tetrahedron Letters, 9 (1971).
58. A.K. Chen and R.W. Woody, J. Amer. Chem. Soc., 93, 29 (1971).
59. P.W. Atkins, Chem. in Britain, 7, 244 (1971).
60. D.J. Caldwell and H. Eyring, Rev. Mod. Phys., 35, 577 (1963).
61. I. Tinoco, Adv. Chem. Phys., 4, 113 (1962).
62. D.J. Caldwell and H. Eyring, The Theory of Optical Activity, Wiley-Interscience, Inc., New York (1971).

II. ORD AND CD OF ORGANIC FUNCTIONAL GROUPS

II-1. Classification of chromophores.

The ORD and CD techniques can be applied to any chromophoric containing optically active compound giving rise to a measurable Cotton effect. This includes natural occurring as well as synthetic (resolved) substances belonging to such fields as terpenes, steroids, carotenoids, lignans, alkaloids, antibiotics, flavonoids, amino acids, peptides, proteins, prostaglandins, carbohydrates, nucleosides, porphyrins, ligands, organometallic compounds, vitamins, human, insect, and plant hormones, etc.

The Cotton effect exhibited by a molecule is associated with the presence of a chromophore (light absorbing group), which is either chiral or in which the dissymmetric vicinity makes the transition optically active. In order to be optically active, the transition must have a non-zero product of electron dipole and magnetic dipole moment: $R_k \neq 0$ in equation [6]. The chromophores can be divided into three main types which sometimes overlap. First, the inherently dissymmetric chromophores, which include non-planar aromatic substances and twisted conjugated systems. Second, the coupled oscillators formed by two non-conjugated chromophores, such as homo-conjugated dienes, non-conjugated arylketones (leading to charge-transfer and orbital-overlap), compounds containing two non-conjugated aromatic amide or peptide chromophores, etc. Third, the perturbed symmetrical chromophores, like a double bond, a saturated carbonyl, carboxyl, and aromatic ring, etc. (see Sec. I-6).

The octant rule for saturated ketones was the first significant and successful attempt to correlate the three-dimensional structure of a chiral molecule with its experimental optical properties (22). More recently, a number of new rules have been proposed for the correlation of the stereochemistry with the optical activity, such as various extensions of the original octant rule, sector, and quadrant rules, etc. All these rules attempt to indicate the sign of contributions to the Cotton effect by groupings of a particular type in different regions of the space around the chromophore. The nodal (or boundary) planes or surfaces of these regions fall into two classes. On the one hand, the true symmetry planes of the chromophore or transition, about the nature and position of which there can be no doubt. On the other hand, the other boundaries of sign regions whose position and shape depend on the nature of the chromophore perturbed and of the perturbing group.

Some of these propositions based either on theoretical considerations or purely experimental, are now available for a variety of chromophoric groupings including olefins, saturated and unsaturated carbonyls, conjugated dienes, styrenes, lactones, aromatic systems, azides, as well as numerous derivatives of acids, alcohols, and amines, etc. The optical properties associated with most common functional groups will be discussed briefly in the following sections.

II-2. Halogenoalkanes.

(+)-Bromochlorofluoromethane (2) exhibits optical activity (17). Examination of various halogenated hydrocarbons by ORD and CD (63,64) shows that 2-halogenoalkanes exhibit Cotton effects corresponding to the $n-\sigma^*$ transition of the carbon-halogen bond. 2-Iodobutane, 2-iodopentane, and 2-iodo-octane present a CD maximum in the 250 nm region. Similarly the UV transition of bromoalkanes at ca. 207 nm gives rise to a Cotton effect in optically active compounds.

Secondary alkyl chlorides also show a Cotton effect appearing below 200 nm. Usually, the Cotton effects are negative for compounds of the
(R)-configuration and positive for the (S)-enan-
tiomers in 2-halogenoalkanes (64). A series of
steroid iodides show the expected CD bands at
about 260 nm, the sign of which for the secondary iodides usually agrees with that reported
for alkyl iodides. However, adjacent hetero-
substituents or unsaturation may invert the sign
(64).

II-3. Isolated double bonds.

Substituted mono-olefinic substances display several UV absorption bands around 200 nm.
Usually at least two of these show optical activity when located in a dissymmetric surrounding.
Albeit it is generally agreed that the λ_1 Cotton
effect is connected with a type of $\pi-\pi^*$ ^{1}transi-
tion, there is less certainty about the origin
of the λ_2 Cotton effect (65). The latter has
been ascribed to a perturbed $\pi_x - \pi_x^*$ transition.
The former band has been assigned to a $\pi_x - \pi_y^*$
transition. However, in certain types of olefins
the λ_2 Cotton effect occurs in the region of the
weak long-wavelength UV absorption, which does
not appear to be of the $\pi-\pi^*$ type, but may be
a $\pi-\sigma_\alpha^*$ or a $\sigma_\alpha -\pi^*$ transition (65).

I   II

In a first analysis, the Cotton effect
around 200 nm may be attributed to a dissymmetric chromophore formed by the double-bond carbon atoms and their allylic quasiaxial hydrogens
(66). The double bond chromophore exhibits a

positive Cotton effect when the geometry will be as in I. Conversely, a negative Cotton effect is observed in the case of a negative helix, as in II.

Alternatively, a substituted olefin can be considered as an asymmetrically perturbed, inherently symmetrical chromophore (67). Accordingly, the Cotton effect sign of the principal $\pi_x - \pi_x^*$ transition reflects the chirality about the olefin chromophore through an olefin octant rule, illustrated in Fig. II-1.

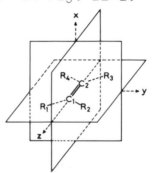

Scott, Wrixon, Tetrahedron, **26**, 3695 (1970)

<u>Fig. II-1.</u>   The octant rule for chiral olefins.

The intersecting symmetry planes of ethylene, being used as octant inferfaces, the olefin is viewed in the z (or -z) direction. The octant signs are derived empirically from the octant location of substituents of several olefins of known absolute configuration and octant diagrams similar to those of the carbonyl group (vide infra). The rule is illustrated in the case of phyllocladene (5a), a diterpenoid olefin. If one looks at molecule (5a) along the z axis (Fig. II-1), one gets the rear octants projection (5b) in which ring A and most of ring B fall into the upper-left octant, thus leading to a negative Cotton effect ($[\theta]_{203}$ -9,800) (Fig. II-2) (67). A more recent analysis of the Cotton effects of substituted olefins considers two categories of cyclohexenes. The first group includes derivatives in which the configuration of the allylic carbon atom appears to determine the sign of the Cotton effect. The second group comprises substituted cyclohexenes in which the conformation of the ring seems to control the sign of the Cotton effect (68,69).

The chiroptical properties of a number of olefins have been reported, including those of trans-cyclooctene, one of the simplest compounds in which the double bond may constitute an inherently dissymmetric chromophore, (see ref. 65-70).

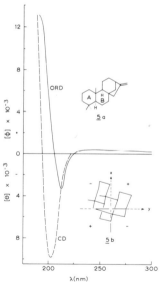

Fig. II-2. The olefin octant rule applied to phyllocladene (5a) (67).

25

Because of the close proximity of the various transitions, the ORD and CD curves of a chiral olefin sometimes consist of a Cotton effect superimposed on a second transition of opposite sign, appearing at a slightly lower wavelength (67–69). Thus, the assignment of absolute stereochemistry of chiral olefins may sometimes require additional verification. In these cases one can use some chromophoric derivative of the double bond to confirm the configuration. Derivatives like osmic esters (71), episulfides (72), thionocarbonates (73), trithiocarbonates (14,72) (see below), organometallic complexes with platinum (74), and the like, have been prepared and their optical properties investigated. This leads to three methods of potential value which may serve for stereochemical assignments of the vicinity of a double bond, namely the study of: a) optically-active intermolecular charge-transfer transition; b) d → d transitions of platinum (II)-olefin complexes; and c) osmate esters (75).

One further important observation germane of the Cotton effects of olefins should be mentioned. The CD properties of the optically active ketone (6a), the olefin (6b), and the phosphorane (6c) have been reported (76). Surprisingly, the low-energy band of the olefin (6b) seems to be devoid of measurable optical activity, although the transition at lower wavelength gives a CD absorption. Similarly, the low-energy transition of the phosphorane (6c) shows no measurable Cotton effect.

$$CH_3\cdots\langle\ \rangle=R$$

6a, R = O
  b, R = C(CH_3)_2
  c, R = P-\varnothing_3

II-4. Dienes.

Theoretical studies of the optical rotatory strength of non-planar butadiene have appeared (43,55). This system is characterized by C_2 symmetry and is thus an inherently chiral entity.

An analysis of the Cotton effect associated with 1,3-cyclohexadienes indicates that the chirality imposed on such diene systems by structural and/or steric factors constitutes an important element of dissymmetry responsible for the Cotton effect. The helicity rule for skewed dienes shown in Fig. II-3, states that a strong positive Cotton effect associated with the lowest frequency cisoid diene $\pi-\pi*$ absorption band, around 260-280 nm in polycyclic substances, indicates that the diene chromophore is twisted in the form of a right-handed helix. Conversely, a strong negative Cotton effect is indicative of a left-handed twist (43,77).

The rule is illustrated in the case of the tetracyclic amine (7) which displays an intense positive Cotton effect (a +1150), in agreement with the right-handed helix formed by the cisoid diene chromophore. Conversely, the diene (8), which forms a left-handed helix, shows an intense negative molecular amplitude (a -244) (14).

7

8

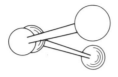   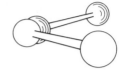

Right - Handed Helix   Left - Handed Helix
Positive Cotton Effet   Negative Cotton Effect

Moscowitz, Charney, Weiss, Ziffer, J. A. C. S., **83**, 4661 (1961).

<u>Fig. II-3.</u>   The helicity rule for skewed dienes.

        Although, formally an inherently dissym-
metric chromophore, expected to exhibit an intense rotational strength, several homo-annular
dienes show rather weak Cotton effects (78,79).
This indicates that the magnitude of the Cotton
effect does not necessarily reflect the intrinsic nature of the chromophore under investigation.   A similar observation has been made in
the case of other chromophores, such as the styrene group, as well as the dimedone and dihydroresorcinol derivatives of amines (see below).
        Numerous optically active dienes follow
the helicity rule, which seems of rather general applicability, provided that there is no interference of other factors such as conformation
and nature of substituents on the diene chromophore or in its vicinity (78,79).   In fact, it
has been shown (53) that configuration interaction among butadiene excitation introduces
cross terms, which substract from the pure configuration strength near an s-<u>cis</u>-geometry.
This may account for the unexpected Cotton effects observed with two skewed dienes belonging

28

to the pentacyclic steroid series (80a). Recently, it was noted that several compounds incorporating one or more oxygen substituents allylic to the diene system, exhibit Cotton effects at variance with the sign predicted by the
helicity rule. It was assumed that the helicity
of the system $O-C-C=C$ may have a larger influence on the CD than the conjugated diene chromophore (80b).

It may be appropriate to mention here
that one has shown that a $5\beta,6\beta$-cyclopropyl Δ^9-
steroid, in which the chirality of the homoan-
nular chromophore corresponds to a left-handed
twist, exhibits an intense negative Cotton ef-
fect. Conversely, a $5\beta,10\beta$-cyclopropyl Δ^6-ste-
roid, in which the conjugated chromophore draws
a right-handed helix, displays a strong positive
molecular amplitude in the same spectral region
(80c).

The allylic axial chirality approach (65,
81) leads to correct sign predictions in the
case of heteroannular cisoid dienes. This approach considers asymmetric perturbations of the
double bond components of the chromophore
through excited-state interactions with their allylic axial or pseudoaxial bonds as the primary
factor controlling the sign of the Cotton effect
(81).

Several transoid dienes have been examined by optical methods (82), and a chirality
rule unfortunately suffering exceptions has been
proposed. The optical properties of some homo-
conjugated dienes (83), and conjugated trienes
(65) have been commented upon.

II-5. Allenes.

According to the Lowe-Brewster rule, the
absolute configuration of chiral allenes is related to the sign of its optical rotation at the
sodium D-line (84). The CD spectra of various
chiral allenes with an established configuration
has led to a bifurcated-quadrant rule, which relates the stereochemistry of the allene chromophore to the sign of the Cotton effect asso-

ciated with the lowest-energy absorption band between 220 and 250 nm (85).

The allene chromophore has four singly-excited $\pi\pi^*$ configurations, resulting from the one-electron promotions, $\pi_x \rightarrow \pi_y^*$, $\pi_y \rightarrow \pi_x^*$, $\pi_x \rightarrow n_x^*$ and $\pi_n \rightarrow n_y^*$, where the xz and yz planes are, respectively, those of the set of bonds to the 1- and to the 3-carbon atom. The antisymmetric combination of the first two configurations gives an excited state to which an electronic transition from the ground state is magnetic-dipole allowed with z-polarization, $A_1 \rightarrow A_2$ in the group D_{2d} of the allene chromophore. The analogous combination of the latter two configurations give an excited state to which a transition from the ground state, $A_1 \rightarrow B_2$, is electric-dipole allowed with z-polarization. A transition to the state formed by the symmetric combination of the former two configurations, B_1, or of the latter two, A_1, has only an electric quadrupole moment (85).

Theoretical treatments of the electronic spectrum of allene place generally the excited $\pi\pi^*$ states in the energy-order, $B_2 > B_1 > A_2$, the position of the A_1 state being variable.

The lowest-energy transition is expected to be magnetic-dipole allowed, $A_1 \rightarrow A_2$, in agreement with the data of Fig. II-4 showing that the lowest-energy CD band of chiral allenes has a dissymmetry factor, $g = \Delta\varepsilon/\varepsilon$, which is relatively large ($g \sim 0.01$). The high intensity of the absorption of alkyl-substituted allenes near 180 nm (see Fig. II-4) suggests that the electric-dipole $A_1 \rightarrow B_2$ transition lies in this region.

A regional rule connecting the position of substituents with the sign of the lowest-energy CD band of a chiral allene is provided by either a static or a dynamic coupling mechanism (85).

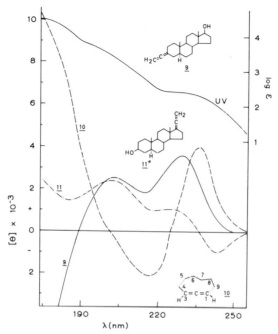

<u>Fig. II-4.</u>   CD curves of the 3-allenyl andro-
stane (<u>9</u>), and of its 17-allenyl isomer (<u>11</u>), CD
and UV curves of (R)-(+)-1,2-cyclononadiene (<u>10</u>)
(85).

       In the dynamic case the magnetic moment
of the $A_1 \rightarrow A_2$ allene transition couples with a
transient electric dipole induced in the substituent by the radiation field to produce optical
activity. The coupling is mediated by the
Coulombic potential between the induced electric
dipole of the substituent and the leading electric multipole of the $A_1 \rightarrow A_2$ allene transition,
the latter being an xyz octupole. If the polarisability of the substituent is isotropic, or if
the contribution of the mean polarisability is
dominant, the regional rule is given by the geometric factor, $XY(7Z^2-R^2)$, for the potential between the z-component of a dipole and the xyz-
component of an octupole.

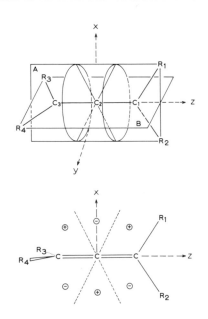

Crabbé, Velarde, Anderson, Clark, Moore, Drake, Mason.
Chem. Comm. 1261 (1971).

Fig. II-5. The bifurcated quadrant rule for chiral allenes. The signs refer to the lowest-energy Cotton effect associated with groups substituted into the +Y hemisphere. The signs are opposite for groups substituted into the -Y hemisphere.

The bifurcated quadrant rule, $XY(7Z^2-R^2)$, shown in Fig. II-5, is consistent with the CD data for chiral allenes in the 220-250 nm region. The CD band of the 3-steroidal allene (9) and of (R)-(+)-1,2-cyclononadiene (10) near 230 nm are comparable in magnitude (Fig. II-4), since the C_6-C_7 bond of (10) lies in the region where $(7Z^2-R^2)$ is negative and the C_4-C_5 and C_8-C_9 bonds in the region where that function is positive. In addition, the CD bands due to the two transitions near 235 and 185 nm, respectively, are of opposite sign for the steroidal allenes (9) and (11), but they have the same sign in the case of (10) (Fig. II-4).

32

Although accessible only to 185 nm the Cotton effect due to the $A_1 \rightarrow B_2$ allene transition is evidently large and Drude plots (equation [2]) of the ORD indicate that it makes the major contribution to the optical rotation at the sodium D-line. In the dynamic coupling mechanism the rotational strength (equation [6]) of the $A_1 \rightarrow B_2$ allene transition depends upon the steric disposition of the substituents and the anisotropy of their polarisabilities, an isotropic group making no contribution. Whilst the C-H bond has a virtually isotropic polarisability, that of the C-C bond is markedly anisotropic, so that the major component of a dipole induced in a C-C bond lies along the bond direction. For (R)-(-)-1,3-dimethyl allene, and other (R)-(-)-substituted allenes, the particular phase-relationship between the induced dipoles of the two C-C bonds from the 1- and 3-carbon atom of the allene chromophore, due to Coulombic interaction with the $A_1 \rightarrow B_2$ transition dipole, gives that transition a negative rotational strength. The D-line optical rotation is consequently negative, in accord with the Lowe-Brewster rule (84).

(R)-(+)-1,2-cyclononadiene (10) contravenes the Lowe-Brewster rule, but the phase-relationships between the induced dipoles along each C-C bond are now such that the $A_1 \rightarrow B_2$ allene transition has an overall positive rotational strength. Whilst the induced dipoles along C_3-C_4 and C_1-C_9 of (10) give a negative contribution, those along $C_5-C_6-C_7-C_8$ coupled with the $A_1 \rightarrow B_2$ transition dipole along $C_1-C_2-C_3$ give a substantially larger positive rotational strength.

The bifurcated quadrant rule has the feature of providing reasonable support for the experimental Cotton effect observed in numerous molecules containing an optically active propadiene chromophore (86).

II-6. Alcohols.

The hydroxyl group is a function absorbing
at low wavelength not accesible to presently
available ORD and CD instruments. Hence, one
can take advantage of the plain ORD curve to assign the configuration to a secondary or tertiary hydroxyl. Whereas 17β-hydroxy-5α-androstane
exhibits a plain positive ORD curve, its 17α-
isomer shows a plain negative curve (14). Plain
ORD curves have also been observed for isomeric
allylic secondary alcohols as well as for tertiary hydroxyl groups (14).

Since the correct configuration will be
more safely deduced from Cotton effect curves
than from plain ORD curves, often one will refer
to chromophoric derivatives of alcohols. For example, the Cotton effect ORD and CD curves of the
2-isothiocyanato derivative of D- and L-2-amino-
butanol methyl carbonate have been obtained.
Both enantiomers exhibit three Cotton effects of
increasing intensity from 350 nm to 200 nm. The
antipodal relationship between the D- and L-iso-
mers is reflected in the mirror-image CD and ORD
curves (87).

The CD data of cuprammonium complexes of
diols and amino-alcohols have been reported (88).
The relationship between the conformation of the
chelate ring and the sign of the Cotton effect
can be used to determine the nature of the cuprammonium complexes of some acyclic ligands, particularly of carbohydrate derivatives. In this respect, it should be mentioned that the ORD and
CD properties of sugar hydrates and various derivatives have been used for stereochemical assignments (89). For example, the molybdate complexes of sugars are suitable for conformational
analysis since they exhibit various CD maxima
between 210 and 350 nm (90). If one pyranose
conformation of a sugar presents three hydroxyls
on its first three carbon atoms in axial-equato-
rial-axial cis-configuration, its molybdate complex displays four Cotton effects in the 220-350
nm region. Conversely, if the hydroxyls on car-

bon atoms 2 and 3 are in the <u>trans</u>-configuration,
the molybdate complex of hexose and pentose al-
dehydic sugars exhibits only two Cotton effects
of opposite sign (90).
      The aromatic chirality method (see Sec.
II-14-c) has been successfully applied to α-
glycols and carbohydrates (91). An extension of
this method has been reported recently (92). It
involves measurement of the CD spectra of α-
glycols in presence of Pr (DPM)$_3$ and Eu (DPM)$_3$
The chirality of the glycol moiety is defined as
being negative or positive respectively, when
the Newman projection represents an anticlockwise
(left-handedness) or clockwise (right-handedness)
rotation from one hydroxyl group to the other.
Mixtures of the glycol and complex lead to CD
curves having two Cotton effects of opposite
signs around 310 and 290 nm. The sign of the
longer wavelength Cotton effect is in agreement
with the chirality of the cyclic α-glycol, as in
the dibenzoate chirality method (92).

11-7. <u>Saturated ketones and aldehydes</u>.

      The weak UV absorption band at ca. 290-
300 nm, associated with the saturated carbonyl
group consists in the promotion of one electron
from a nonbonding $2p_y$ orbital of the oxygen atom
to an antibonding orbital involving both the carbon and the oxygen atoms of the carbonyl group
(n-π* transition). Theoretical treatments of
the origin of Cotton effects and the symmetry
rules relating the sign and magnitude of a Cotton effect to the geometry of the dissymmetric
surroundings of a symmetrical chromophore have
led to some controversy. The present theoretical situation seems to indicate that the three
mechanisms which have been proposed to explain
the origin of optical activity, <u>i.e.</u>, the one-
electron mechanism, the coupling of two electric
transition moments, and the coupling of one electric and one magnetic moment, should be considered as complementary and not as alternatives
(44).

The experimental data accumulated on the Cotton effect associated with the saturated carbonyl chromophore have led to the proposition of the octant rule (22), which establishes the absolute stereochemistry from the sign and intensity of the Cotton effect. Conversely, the sign of the Cotton effect can be predicted from the stereochemistry around the carbonyl.

In the original rule, the carbonyl being the reference point, a cyclohexanone is divided into octants by three mutually perpendicular planes. These are nodal and symmetry planes of the orbitals involved in the n-π* transition of the carbonyl (12,14,15). This concept is not limited to the cyclohexanone ring (22), but is applicable to cyclobutanone (93), cyclopentanone (76,94), cycloheptanone (95), i.e., to any ring system or aliphatic chain carrying a carbonyl grouping (14).

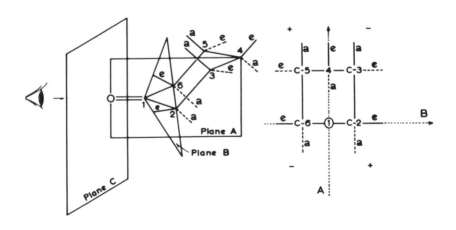

Moffitt, Woodward, Moscowitz, Klyne, Djerassi, J. A. C. S., **83**, 4013 (1961).

Fig. II-6.   The octant rule for the carbonyl chromophore.

In Fig. II-6, plane A is vertical and passes through carbon atoms C-1 and C-4. The only substituents in plane A are attached to C-4. The horizontal plane B encompasses the carbon atom possessing the carbonyl (C-1) and its two adjacent carbon atoms (C-2 to the right and C-6 to the left). The substituents equatorially oriented, attached to these carbon atoms (C-2 and C-6), lie nearly in the nodal plane B. Planes A and B provide four octants: the back octants, shown in Fig. II-6. A third plane, C, perpendicular to A and dissecting the oxygen-carbon atom (C-1) bond, produces four additional octants, called front octants.

According to the octant rule (22) substituents lying in planes A and B make no contribution to the Cotton effect of the carbonyl. This includes the equatorial substituents on C-2 and C-6, provided that they are exactly in the plane, as well as both substituents on C-4. In addition, the atoms or groupings situated in an axial configuration on C-2 (lower-right octant) and the axial and equatorial substituents on C-5 (upper-left octant) make a positive contribution to the Cotton effect. Conversely, substituents situated in an axial configuration on C-6 (lower-left octant), as well as the axial and equatorial substituents on C-3 lead to a negative Cotton effect.

An illustration of this rule is provided by 5α-cholestan-3-one (12a) which displays a positive Cotton effect (a +56; [θ] +4,200) around 300 nm. In fact, the octant projection of this substance indicates that carbon atoms C-6, C-7, C-15, and C-16 lie in positive octants. Conversely, in coprostan-3-one, which is the 5β-isomer (12b), carbon atoms C-6, C-7, C-15, and C-16 make a negative contribution to the Cotton effect, thus both the molecular amplitude (a -27) and the molecular ellipticity ([θ] -1,500) are negative.

The Kronig-Kramers theorem (25,50,96) leads to an expression [7] which relates semiquantitatively the molecular amplitude of the

ORD curve to the dichroic absorption of the corresponding CD curve of a saturated ketone:

[7] $a = 40.28 \cdot \Delta\epsilon$

In terms of molecular ellipticity $[\theta]$, equation [7] becomes [8]:

[8] $a = 0.0122 \cdot [\theta]$

By applying equation [8] to D-(+)-camphor (1) one obtains: a = 0.0122.+5,115 = +62; a +64 is the experimental result from the ORD curve in Fig. I-2.

Similarly, when equation [8] is applied to steroids (12a) and (12b) one also finds a good agreement between the ORD and CD values.

Although, expressions [7] and [8] are very useful, it should be emphasized that they were obtained for the n-π* transition of a saturated carbonyl and must be used with caution for other chromophores.

For twisted or skewed molecules, such as cyclopentanone derivatives (e.g. 17-keto steroids), or twisted cyclohexanones, etc., one should distinguish between first-order and second-order effects. The first-order effects are attributed to the skewed carbon atoms of the ring system itself. The second-order effects are due to the substituents. However, second-order effects are generally overwhelmed by first-order effects of the ring system. For instance, if one applies the octant rule to the cyclohexanone formed by carbon atoms 8, 9, 11, 12, 15, and 16 of the diterpenic derivative (13), the experimental Cotton effect ($[\theta]_{302}$ -6740) is in agreement with the octant projection (13a). Indeed, carbon atom C-9 is strongly skewed in a negative octant. The negative contribution of C-9 is assisted by the fact that ring A is also located in a negative octant, whilst C-14 is situated in a positive octant (97).

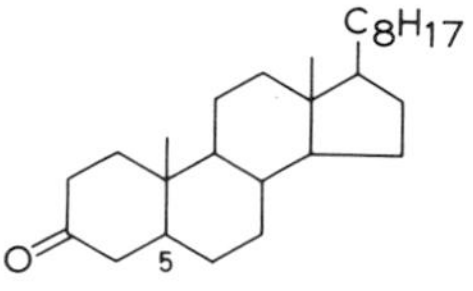

12 a, 5αH
   b, 5βH

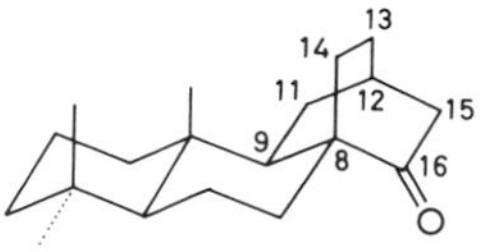

13

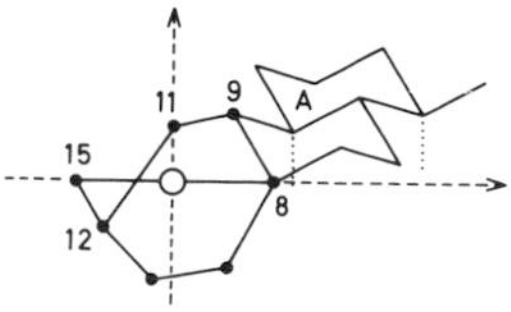

13 a

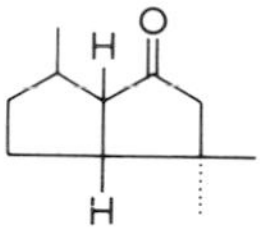

14

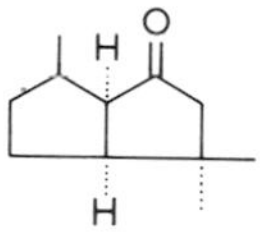

15

The strong Cotton effect exhibited by the bicyclic ketones (14) and (15) is mainly due to the skewed carbon atoms of the cyclopentanone ring. The cis-β-bicyclic ketone (14) exhibits an intense positive CD curve ($[\theta]_{301}$ +11,350), whereas the cis α isomer (15) presents a negative CD curve of strong intensity ($[\theta]_{302}$ -11,520) (98). A similar explanation accounts for the positive Cotton effect shown by D-(+)-camphor (1) (Fig. I-2).

The next example shows that sometimes the preferred conformation of a molecule can be deduced from the sign of the Cotton effect. The 9-methyl-cis-1-decalone (16a) can adopt either the chair conformation (16b) or (16c). According to the octant rule, this bicyclic ketone would present a negative or a positive Cotton effect respectively, in the two possible two-chair conformations (16b) and (16c). In fact, the experimental Cotton effect is positive (a +51), indicating that the molecule chooses the preferred conformation (16c). One concludes that if the absolute configuration of a ketonic compound is known, its absolute conformation can be assigned on the basis of its Cotton effect. Conversely, if the conformation of a substance is established, one can deduce its absolute configuration from its optical properties (see Fig. II-7).

16a   16 b   16 c

Table II-1, listing the Cotton effect associated with the saturated carbonyl group located in various positions of the steroid nucleus is a good illustration of the usefulness of the chiroptical properties for the assignment of both structure and stereochemistry (14).

In spite of some relatively minor but pertinent questions (45,46,99), well over a thousand papers have now been published on successful applications of the octant rule for all classes of optically active compounds, from ketone-containing aliphatic substances to polycyclic molecules (14).

II-8.   α-Cyclopropyl, α-epoxyketones, vicinal effects.

A "reversed" octant rule has been proposed for α-cyclopropyl and α-epoxyketones (100). An illustration of the "inverted" octant rule is provided by the comparison of the Cotton effect exhibited by 3-methylcyclohexanone (17; [θ] +1980) and 6-methyl [2:5]-spiro 4-octanone (18; [θ] +960) (101). The original octant rule would predict a substantial increase of the positive

Table II-1 Cotton Effect of Keto Steroids (14)

Position of the carbonyl group	Configuration	Cotton Effect	
		ORD Molecular amplitude a	CD Molecular ellipticity [θ]
1	5αH	− 25	− 1,200
	5βH	− 136	− 11,100
2	5αH	+ 120	+ 9,800
	5βH	− 34	− 2,800
3	5αH	+ 56	+ 4,200
	5βH	− 27	− 1,500
4	5αH	− 94	− 7,700
	5βH	+ 3	+ 250
6	5αH	− 76	− 4,600
	5βH	− 160	− 14,000
7	5αH	− 23	− 2,200
	5βH	+ 29	+ 2,400
11	5αH	+ 13	+ 1,100
	5βH	+ 15	+ 1,230
12	5αH	+ 40	+ 3,300
	5βH	+ 20	+ 1,900
15	14αH	+ 140	+ 11,000
	14βH	100	− 8,200
16	14αH	− 240	− 19,000
	14βH	+ 137	+ 11,200
17	14αH	+ 140	+ 11,400
	14βH	+ 34	+ 3,500

Cotton effect in going from (17) to (18), since
the cyclopropane ring is located on carbon atom
C-2 in Fig. II-6. Instead, the molecular ellipticity of (18) is less than half that of (17),
showing the negative contribution of the cyclo-
propyl ring.

17   18   21

        Some exceptions of this rule have been
reported (102). A careful CD investigation of
numerous such ketones has shown that the sign of
the π–π* Cotton effect is dictated by the octant
in which the methylene group (in cyclopropyl-
ketones) or oxygen group (in epoxy-ketones) lies.
The sign follows the normal and reversed octant
rules respectively (103).
        The unexpected chiroptical properties ex-
hibited by some α-epoxy and α-cyclopropyl-ketones
indicate that caution should be exercised when
applying the octant rule to ketones which have a
functional group in the vicinity of the carbonyl
(99,102,103). In fact, it has been shown that
α-fluoro-ketones (12,14), some hydroxy-ketones
(14), α-ketols, α-acetoxy-ketones (104), as well
as amino-ketones (105), sometimes display Cotton
effects which do not obey the original octant
rule. The fact that caution should be exercised
before applying simple rules to molecules presenting unusual electronic patterns is further
illustrated in the case of β, γ -cyclopropyl
ketones for which neither the octant rule nor reversed octant rules correctly predict the sign
of the Cotton effect in all cases studied (106).

II-9. α,β-Unsaturated ketones.

Conjugated ketones show at least two absorption maxima between 220 and 400 nm. The intense UV maximal absorption between 230 and 260 nm is associated with the $\pi-\pi^*$ transition (K band) of the conjugated carbonyl group. The less intense absorption band around 340 nm corresponds to the $n-\pi^*$ carbonyl transition (R-band). Both transitions are optically active in an asymmetric surrounding.

Fig. II-7 reproduces the CD curve of a pair of enantiomeric diketo-steroids (19a) and (19b) (107). The mp, UV, IR, NMR, and MS properties of these isomers are identical. Their optical properties allowed to confirm their relative and absolute configuration. Fig. II-7 shows that both transitions of the Δ^4-3-keto-chromophore are optically active, but a more intense optical activity is associated with the K band than with the R band which presents a multiple Cotton effect at ca. 340 nm. Since the ORD and CD curves of (19a) and (19b) are mirror images, one concludes that these compounds are indeed enantiomers, thus establishing their relative configuration. Moreover, because Δ^4-3-keto-steroids of known 9α,10β-absolute configuration, such as testosterone (20), exhibit a negative Cotton effect in the 340 nm region and an intense positive Cotton effect around 250 nm, ipso facto, by correlation the absolute stereochemistry of the steroid (19a) and hence of its enantiomer (19b) can be assigned (107).

In α,β-unsaturated ketones one or both orthogonal reflection planes are lost, so that the octant rule is in general no longer applicable in its original form. Extensions of the octant rule have been proposed for the $n-\pi^*$ transition of conjugated ketones (108).

The enone chirality rule states that the sign of the $n-\pi^*$ transition of conjugated transoid enones follows an inverse octant rule (108).

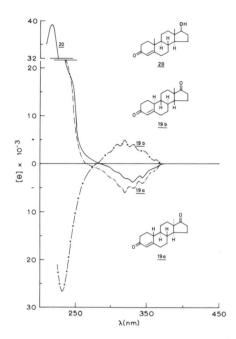

Fig. II-7. CD curves of steroids (19a), (19b), and (20) (107).

This proposition, which does not apply to cyclopentenones, seems to account for numerous experimental data, but should be used with caution (109). The assignment of the β-configuration to the 14-methyl in stachysterone A (21) constitutes an elegant application of this rule (110). The sign of the enone n-π* Cotton effect centered around 346 nm is negative in (21), and opposite to that of other ecdysones. In view of the relationship of n-π* Cotton effect signs to the enone chirality (108), this indicates that in stachysterone A (21) the 6-one and 7-ene are twisted in a clockwise sense, thus confirming the stereochemistry at C-14 to be β (110).

The π-π* transition of conjugated enones usually exhibits a Cotton effect of opposite sign to that of the R-band (111). However, a careful examination of the ORD and CD curves of a number of α,β-unsaturated ketones revealed the presence of a new strong optically active band close to the $\pi-\pi^*$ transition (112). As a result, the sign of the Cotton effect associated with the K band observed by ORD is sometimes obscured by this overlapping near transition. In addition, a fourth CD band presumably due to a $\pi-\sigma^*$ transition, usually of high intensity, has been detected at <u>ca</u>. 210 nm (113a).

Table II-2

Cotton Effect of Steroidal Enones in the 200-220 nm Region (81)

Conjugated keto-steroids	α'-Chirality contribution	Experimental Cotton effect
4-En-3-one	$2\beta H$ (+)	+
B-Nor-4-en-3-one	$2\beta H$ (+)	+
5-En-4-one	$3\alpha H$ (−)	−
4-En-6-one	$7\alpha H$ (+)	+
5-En-7-one	$8\beta H$ (−)	−
8(9)-En-7-one	$6\beta H$ (+)	+
8(14)-En-7-one	$6\beta H$ (+)	+
8(9)-En-11-one	$12\alpha H$ (−)	−
9(11)-En-12-one	$13\beta Me$ (+)	+

When applied to cyclic conjugated enones, the allylic axial chirality approach suggests that the Cotton effect in the 250 nm region is usually dominated by allylic axial perturbations of the carbon-carbon double bond. According to the same rule, the Cotton effect at <u>ca</u>. 210 nm reflects the chirality contribution to the car-

bonyl group by the pseudoaxial bond on the α'
carbon (65,81). This is illustrated in Table
II-2 in the case of some steroidal enones. Finally, the chiroptical properties of Δ^4-3-keto-
steroids may be rationalized in terms of the
contributions of the pseudoaxial bonds on the α'
and γ carbon atoms (113b).

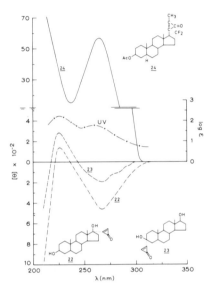

Fig. II-8. CD and UV curves of the cyclopro-
penonyl steroids (22), (23), and (24).

      The cyclopropenone can be considered as
the smallest cyclic α,β-unsaturated keto-system.
The UV spectrum of the 17α-cyclopropenonyl-andro-
stane derivative (22) (114) shows a transition at
259 nm which is optically active and presents a
negative Cotton effect (Fig. II-8). In addition,
a weakly positive Cotton effect is observed at
227 nm. A negative Cotton effect is associated
with the 3α-cyclopropenonyl group in (23), whilst
the 17β-cyclopropenonyl steroid (24) exhibits a
positive Cotton effect (79). The CD Cotton effect of the 17α-cyclopropenonyl derivative (22)
is more intense than that of its 3α-isomer (23).

This can be attributed to steric factors, which leave less conformational freedom to the 17α-cyclopropenone chromophore than at C-3. Similarly, the 17β-cyclopropenonyl steroid (24) presents a more intense Cotton effect than the isomers (22) or (23), because of the frozen conformation of the 17β-side chain in (24). It is of interest to note that the signs of the Cotton effect associated with the 265 nm transition in these 17α- (22) (see Fig. II-8) and 17β-cyclopropenonyl (24) steroids are the same as in the corresponding 17-acetyl (methyl ketone) steroids (14).

The optical properties of some α,β-epoxyenones have been reported recently and reliance of the sign of the Cotton effects to the chirality of the chromophore has been established (115).

II-10. β,γ-Unsaturated ketones.

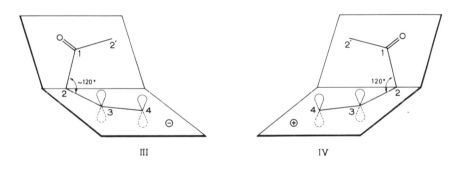

III   IV

Moscowitz, Mislow, Glass, Djerassi, J.A.C.S., 84, 1945 (1962).

If the geometry is appropriate in β,γ-unsaturated ketones, the nonbonding n-electrons on the carbonyl oxygen interact with the π-electrons of the homoconjugated ethylene-carbonyl π-system (32,39). Hence, in a variety of β,γ-unsaturated ketones the n-π* transition borrows intensity from the allowed π-π* transition, with concomitant enhancement of the extinction coefficient of the ultraviolet 300 nm band and the rotatory power (36,116). This indicates that the β,γ-unsaturated carbonyl system constitutes an inherently dissymmetric chromophore. A modification of the octant rule proposed for this chromophore suggests that the chirality of the β,γ-unsaturated keto chromophore may be discussed in terms of the geometric representations III. and IV (36, 116).

Two planes are defined by $C_2'-C_1^{\overset{O}{=}}-C_2$ and $C_2-C_3-C_4$ portions of the chromophore which intersect at a dihedral angle greater than 90° (about 120° in rigid structures). As indicated in III and IV, the arrangement $C_2'-C_1^{\overset{O}{=}}-C_2-C_3-C_4$ assumes one of two enantiomeric conformations, one giving rise to (III), a negative, and the other to (IV), a positive Cotton effect (36,116).

The very strong positive Cotton effect exhibited by the diterpene ($\underline{25}$; $[\theta]_{304}$ +37,750) is in agreement with geometry IV for the β,γ-unsaturated keto-chromophore (97).

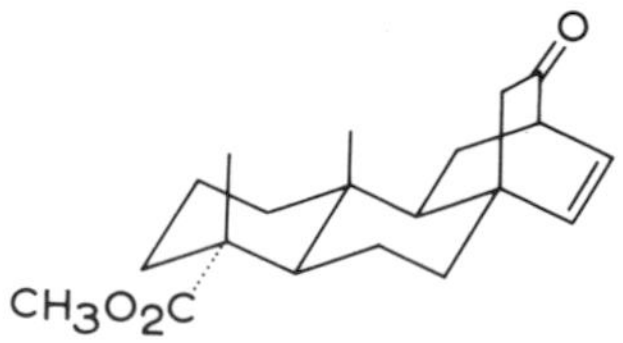

$\underline{25}$

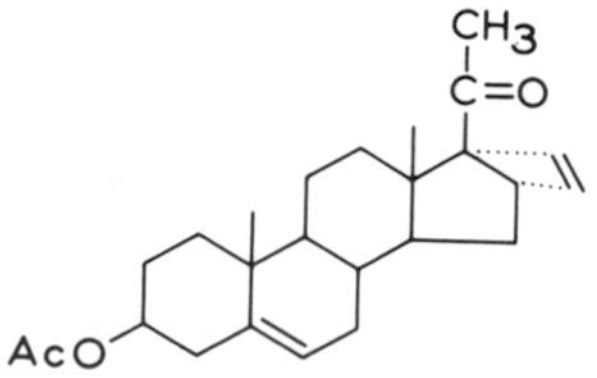

$\underline{26}$

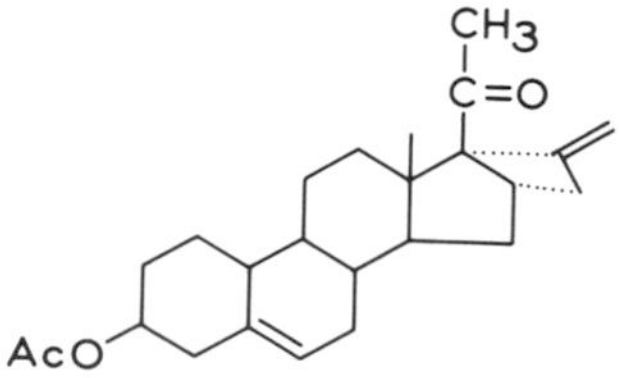

$\underline{27}$

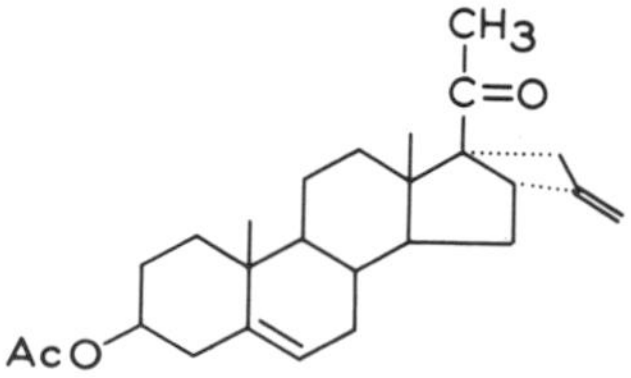

$\underline{28}$

The pentacyclic steroids (26), (27), and (28) exhibit respectively a strong positive (26; $[\Theta]_{300}$ +15,380) an intense negative (27; $[\Theta]_{295}$ -18,180), and a positive (28; $[\Theta]_{295}$ +5,780), Cotton effect. The examination of the geometry of the homoconjugated system with molecular models, indicates compound (26) to correspond to geometry IV, whereas the β,γ-unsaturated chromophore of the steroid (27) has a conformation similar to III (117). Finally, in agreement with its structure and stereochemistry, the exomethylene isomer (28) presents the weakly positive Cotton effect, typical of the 17α-substituted 20-keto-steroids (14).

As shown above, in some molecules unsaturated chromophores not directly bound to one another are nevertheless sufficiently close in space for their electron clouds to interact. This intramolecular interaction then leads to changes relative to the absorption of separated chromophores, even though the chromophoric groups are not conjugated in the classical sense. Such a situation is encountered in some aromatic 11-keto-steroids.

CD has allowed a detailed study of both the configuration and conformation of the aromatic keto-steroids (29a), (29b), and (30a), (30b) (118). Although the classical UV properties of these compounds are rather similar, the inversion of configuration at C-9, in going from the 9α-steroid (29a; $[\Theta]$ +9,000) to its 9β-isomer (29b; $[\Theta]$ +50,200), is accompanied by a substantial increase of the Cotton effect. Examination of the geometry of these systems with molecular models indicates that in (29b) the arrangement of the 11-carbonyl group vis-a-vis the aromatic A-ring is similar to conformation IV. Hence, the very strong Cotton effect of (29b) can be interpreted in terms of homoconjugation between the carbonyl and benzene π-electrons. The difference of positive Cotton effects exhibited by (29b) and (30b; $[\Theta]$ +26,700) is attributed to a boat conformation of ring C in (30b) to reduce 1-methyl-11-keto interactions, whilst it is a chair in (29b). In

both compounds (29b) and (30b) the aromatic ring
falls into a positive octant, indicating that
these aromatic β-keto-steroids follow the classical octant rule.

A detailed study of the absorption and
chiroptical properties of 3-exo- and 3-endo-
phenyl-2-norbornanone revealed only a slight enhancement of the carbonyl n-π* transition due to
α-phenyl substitution (119). The contribution
of the α-phenyl groupings to the n-π* transition
cannot be rationalized on the basis of back octant effects, but can be understood on the basis
of transition moment coupling or front octant
effects (119). In this respect it is worth men-
tioning that besides antioctant behavior (46,99),
front octant effects have been reported on various occasions (120).

29 a, 9α H
   b, 9β H

30 a, 9β H
   b, 9αH

In summary, the n-π* Cotton effects of
non-conjugated ketones are usually low as in saturated carbonyls, intermediate as in axial α-
haloketones, twisted systems, cyclopentanones,
or high as in some β,γ-unsaturated ketones and
in β-aryl-ketones, depending upon the extent to
which the asymmetrically perturbing orbitals mix
with the orbitals of the carbonyl grouping.

II-11. Carboxylic acids, esters, lactones,
       lactams, imides, anhydrides.

Optically active acids, esters, and related groups present a Cotton effect in the 210
nm region, attributed to the n-π* transition of
the carboxyl. Semi-empirical rules have been

proposed for the Cotton effects associated with such chromophores (121-126). For simple acids a correlation can be made between the sign of the experimental Cotton effect and the absolute configuration at the single asymmetric carbon atom. For more complex acids of known absolute configuration, the preferred conformations of the carboxyl group have been discussed in terms of a carboxyl sector rule, originally developed for lactones.

The relationship between the conformation and absolute configuration of lactones and the sign and magnitude of long-wavelength Cotton effects leads to a lactone sector rule, which divides the space around the lactone group into sectors by means of planes meeting at the carboxyl carbon atom (121-125). It was suggested that the signs used for the ketone octant rule must be reversed for lactone sectors. Thus, atoms or groups lying in the back upper-right and lower-left sectors make positive contributions to the Cotton effect, whilst atoms in the back upper-left and lower-right sectors contribute negatively to the Cotton effect (Fig. II-9). Each carbon-oxygen bond in the lactone group has some double-bond character, and is considered in turn as a double bond. When diagrams (A) and (B) in Fig. II-9 are superimposed as in (C), the signs of the contributions in some sectors cancel in varying degree, whereas in other sectors the contributions reinforce one another.

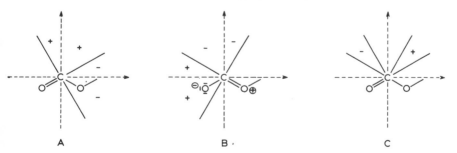

A   B ·   C

Jennings, Klyne, Scopes, J.C.S., 7211, 7229 (1965).

Fig. II-9. The carboxyl sector rule.

If one applies the lactone sector rule to the sesquiterpene derivative (31), two different views of the molecule must be considered. First, a view along the bisectrix of the O-C=O angle (31a), similar to the ordinary ketone octant projection. Second, a view of the molecule from above, projected onto the lactone plane, the new projection (31b). In the case of the eudesmane derivative (31), the lactone sector rule predicts a positive Cotton effect, in agreement with the experimental findings (121).

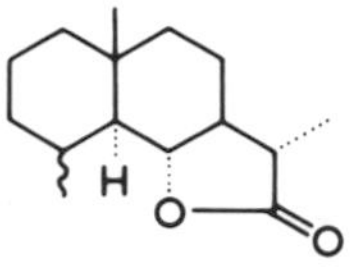

31

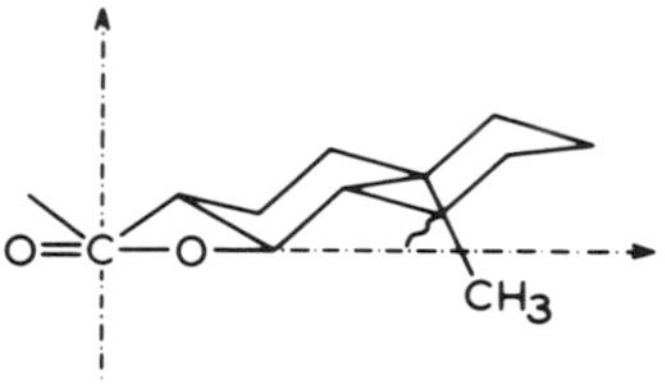

31a 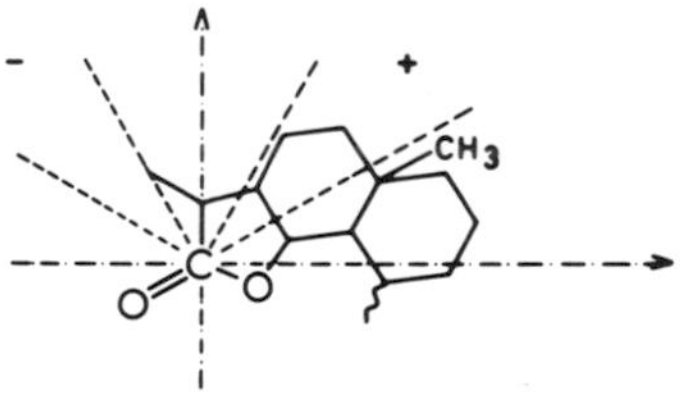   31b

In δ-lactones the optical properties depend on the conformation of the ring. If the chirality of the lactone is established, the sign of its Cotton effect can be deduced. Conversely, from the sign of the Cotton effect, one can ascertain the conformation of the ring system (123). In fact, both the ring-chirality and the configuration of carbon atoms and substituents adjacent (Cα,Cβ) to the chromophore should be considered (124). In γ-lactones the Cotton effect depends mainly upon the location of Cβ relative to the planar lactone system (125). The situation is similar to that in some bi- and poly-cyclic cyclopentanones, in which the out-of-plane

52

carbon atoms of the five-membered ring have a dominant influence on the Cotton effect of the ketone (see Sec. II-7). Hence, there is some evidence that the Cotton effect associated with the n–π* transition in lactones and lactams is determined both in sign and magnitude by interactions within the asymmetric ring (125).

Although the Cotton effect of the acetate group can be used to establish the configuration of secondary and tertiary hydroxyls, a difficulty results from the fact that usually most of the molecule falls in front sectors, and it is only assumed that substituents in front sectors make contributions opposite to those in back sectors (126).

In carboxylic acids and esters, a significant optical activity indicates an appreciable degree of conformational preference, even though free rotation is formally possible about the carbon-carboxyl bond.

The effect of α-alkyl substitution on the n–π* Cotton effect of some α-chloro and α-bromo alkyl carboxylic acids has been studied (127). In addition, the CD properties of (2 R)-mercaptopropionic acid and related compounds have been reported (128). The n–π* Cotton effects of unsaturated acids have also been reported (129). In conjugated lactones, usually three optically active bands can be detected, which are attributed to an n–π*, and π–σ* transition, respectively (130).

Several dicarboxylic acids have also been investigated (122,131). Monosubstituted succinic acids with the D configuration display positive Cotton effects when the substituent is an alkyl, thioalkyl group, or bromine and chlorine. Conversely, hydroxy acids and amino acids with the same configuration present opposite Cotton effects. In addition, the chiroptical properties of substituted succinic acids, of relatively simple structure are inverted in alkaline medium. The analysis of the chiroptical properties of some trans-dicarboxylic acids allows to decide whether these molecules are fixed in a rigid conformation or if they are flexible systems. Al-

53

though the UV spectra show only the n–π* carboxy-
ylate transition around 210 nm, the ORD and CD
curves are dominated by the π–π* transition,
which appears at 200–203 nm in flexible systems,
but is shifted to 209–210 nm in rigid conformations (131). The red shift supports the hypo-
thesis that the carboxyl groupings are coupled
in the latter molecules (131). This behaviour
predicted by theory has been observed in other
similar instances (132). One concludes that if
an optically active molecule possesses two identical neighboring chromophores, the chiroptical
methods provide a way to test the conformational
rigidity through application of the exciton theory (131,132).

A CD study on the effect of conformational
restriction and rigidity of mono- and bicyclic
lactones has been reported (·133). The experimental results on six-membered-ring dilactones, relative to diketo-piperazines, are in agreement
with similar findings (51) on the behaviour of
five-membered cyclic esters and amides. Moreover
a careful investigation of the CD properties of
bridged lactones in solvents of different polarity is required before any correlation between
the sign of Cotton effects and molecular conformation can be made.

The CD properties of some α,β-cyclopropyl-
lactones have been investigated, and the rule
proposed for cyclopropyl-ketones (Sec. II-8)
seems to be applicable to this chromophore (115,
134). α,β-Epoxy-conjugated lactones have also
been studied (115).

Other derivatives of the carboxyl group
(e.g. carbobenzoxy, tert-butyloxycarbonyl, imide,
phenylimide, anilide, etc.), as well as anhy-
drides of dicarboxylic acids exhibit Cotton effects which reflect the stereochemistry in the
vicinity of the chromophore (14,15,135) (see below).

II-12. α-Hydroxy and α-amino acids.

A considerable effort has been devoted to
the assignment of absolute configuration to a va-

54

riety of α-hydroxy acids (12-15,121,122). In
addition, the interest in the chiroptical properties of α-amino acids is illustrative of the
general attention being given to those small molecules which constitute the building blocks for
biologically important macromolecules (Sec. IV-1,
V-1) (12-15). The carboxyl sector rule (121) is
suitable for the prediction of preferred align-
ments of many amino acids and esters. α-Hydroxy
acids and α-amino acids of L configuration show
a positive Cotton effect around 215 nm, whilst
their D-enantiomers display a Cotton effect of
opposite sign (121,122). Thus, aliphatic amino
acids show a unique Cotton effect, the sign of
which reflects the stereochemistry at the asymmetric center. The exact wavelength where the
carboxyl n-π^* Cotton effect appears, as well as
its intensity vary with the pH of the medium.
The amino acids examined in acid medium present
their ORD first extremum at ca. 225 nm, λ_0 around
210-212 nm, and their second extremum in the
195-200 nm region. The molecular amplitudes depend on the size of the alkyl substituents. L-
alanine, the most symmetric compound investigated
(136), shows the lowest amplitude. Substitution
of the alkyl chain progressively increases the
intensity of the Cotton effect from L-valine to
α-amino butyric acid (14,15,136,137).

Effects related to molecular structure
and to the state of ionization of the species,
using the fully protonated form as reference
states have been observed. One has shown the
influence of vibrational fine structure on the
absorption-CD relation, and some examples of the
utility of comparing the UV, ORD, and CD data
have been reported (137).

Recently, a sector rule has been proposed
which relates the sign and intensity of the Cotton effect with the conformation and absolute
configuration of α-amino acids (138). A careful
structural analysis of α-amino acids has indicated a preferred conformation in solution, in
which the N-C-COO atoms are coplanar. The C-O
bond of the carboxylate ion, or of the unionized
carboxyl group, is cis to the C-N, with the hy-

drogen atoms on the nitrogen staggered with respect to C-O. Because an n-π* transition is involved in the absorption of both the carbonyl
and carboxylate groups, both C-O bonds in the
carboxylate ion may be considered as two equivalent carbonyl groups, separated by 120°. As
indicated in Fig. II-10, the plane bisecting the
carboxylate ion is considered as a symmetry
plane (plane A). If one assigns two additional
planes (P_1 and P_2), through the carboxylate carbon atom, each perpendicular to a C-O bond, and
if one applies the ketone octant rule to each
C-O, one observes cancellation of contributions
in some 30° sectors, and reinforcement in others
(Fig. II-10). This leads to a positive contribution for substituents in a 30° sector in the
center of the upper-right rear quadrant, and a
negative contribution in a 30° sector in the center of the upper-left rear quadrant. Since the
carboxylate ion has a true plane of symmetry,
the corresponding sectors below the plane are of
opposite sign. Sectors of 60° where groups make
no contribution to the optical activity have
their centers on each of the major perpendicular
planes A and B in Fig. II-10.

This rule clearly shows that only the
side chain group and the hydrogen atom attached
to the α-carbon atom make significant contributions to the Cotton effect (138).

A is a symmetry plane bisecting the carboxylate ion. Both planes P_1 and P_2 are perpendicular to each C-O bond. The inner circles
show independent contributions of each C-O by
the ketone octant rule. The substituents making
positive and negative contributions are apparent
on the outer circle.

Amino acids containing other absorbing
groups, like an aromatic ring, lead to multiple
Cotton effect curves (42b,136-139). An ORD
study of a series of derivatives of L-phenylalanine substituted in the aromatic ring indicates
temperature-dependence of the parameters of the
Drude equation (see equation [2]) (139).

56

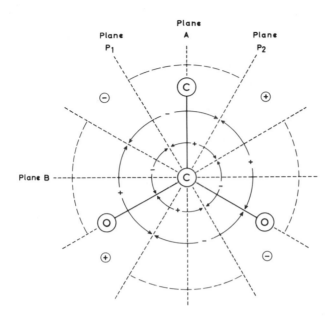

Jorgensen, Tetrahedron Letters, 863 (1971).

Fig. II-10. The carboxylic group viewed from the top in amino acids.

The aromatic amino acids exhibit positive Cotton effects corresponding to the $^1B_{2u} \longleftarrow {}^1A_{1g}$ aromatic electronic transition which has a low rotational strength and which is structure-dependent. The second aromatic transition seems to interfere with the n–π* band of the carboxyl group. The optical properties of β-aryl amino acids outside the region of the Cotton effects are ascribed to the vicinal effect of the aryl substituent. The chromophore most affected by this vicinal effect seems to absorb below 200 nm. An optically active n–σ* transition of the N–C$_\alpha$ bond may be involved. For example, the chiroptical properties of D-phenylglycine and L-phenylalanine measured at various pH, suggest an interaction between the ^1L_a transition of the benzene ring

and the n–π* band of the carboxyl group (139)
(see Sec. II-14).

The ORD and CD of lactic acid and mandel-
ic acid derivatives have been reinvestigated,
and abnormal properties (such as bands at ca.
240 nm) have been reported for conformationally
mobile α-amino acids and α-hydroxy acids. The
apparently aberrant ORD and CD spectra exhibited
by several members of these series seem to be
due to the nucleophilic character of the hetero-
atom attached to the asymmetric center, leading
to the existence of various conformers and/or to
the presence of different structural species in
equilibrium (140,141). Similarly, the CD of D-
(+)-tartaric acid shows a Cotton effect around
255 nm, attributed to an isomeric cyclic structure of the molecule (142).

When the integral Cotton effect of the
carboxyl chromophore cannot be reached easily or
leads to doubtful results, one will refer to derivatives either of the carboxyl group or of the
hydroxyl and amino functions (Sec. II-11, II-16,
II-21) in which the absorption band is shifted
towards higher wavelengths.

Since molybdate complexes of hydroxyls
are easily obtained (90), it was anticipated
that such organo-metallic derivatives of α-hydroxy acids could be formed. In fact these complexes lead to Cotton effect curves which can be
used for stereochemical assignments (143). Similarly, the chiroptical properties of complexes
of nickel (II) (144), complexes of copper (II)
(145), and complexes of triethylenetetramine-co-
balt (III) (146) with amino acids have been reported.

II-13. Oximes.

The oxime of a saturated carbonyl has a
relatively simple UV absorption pattern, which
can easily be investigated by the optical methods. The sign and intensity of the Cotton effects reflect the stereochemistry in the vicinity of the chromophore (14,147).

Whereas α,β-unsaturated ketones exhibit several absorption bands between 350 and 210 nm (see Sec. II-9), the situation is simpler in the case of the corresponding oximes. In fact, the CD curves of steroids (32) and (33) present one major Cotton effect, devoid of fine structure, around 240 nm, (compare with the multiple Cotton effects in Fig. II-7). Similarly, the Cotton effects of dienone-oximes are simpler than those of the corresponding ketones, and their sign also reflects the stereochemistry around the chromophore (14). Hence, sometimes the Cotton effect exhibited by oximes will give safer stereochemical information than in the case of the parent ketones. In some cases it has been noted that the Cotton effects of oximes can be substantially affected by the nature of the solvent (14, 147).

32   33

II-14. Aromatic chromophores.

Most simple aromatic compounds show three absorption bands which become optically active in a dissymmetric surrounding, i.e., the 180-190 nm transition (called β, $'B_a$, $'A_{1g} \rightarrow 'E_{1u}$, $^1A \rightarrow {}^1B$ or E_1), the 200-220 nm band (p, $'L_a$, $'A_{1g} \rightarrow 'B_{1u}$, $^1A \rightarrow {}^1L_a$ or E_2) and the 260-280 nm transition (α, $'L_b$, $'A_{1g} \rightarrow 'B_{2u}$, $^1A \rightarrow {}^1L_b$ or B) (148). In spite of the wealth of optical da-

ta available on aromatic chromophores, theoretical studies are limited to a few groups of compounds. Rules of empirical origin and some
based on theory have been proposed for molecules
containing aromatic chromophores in rigid systems (149) as well as phenyls (42b,44,149,150),
tetrasubstituted phenyls (151), biaryls (116,
152), phenylosotriazoles (153), purines (154),
cyclonucleosides (56), helicenes (31,155), etc.
Recently, in a general approach to the study of
the Cotton effect of aromatic chromophores, a
set of rules for benzene transitions has been
proposed (156). Different propositions have
shown that often one can deduce the stereochemistry, i.e., the absolute configuration of asymmetric centers and the conformation of rings or
conjugated systems from the sign and magnitude
of the Cotton effects.

34   35

The helicity of hexahelicene with a simple inherently dissymmetric chromophore apparently of P configuration (157) was established by
the dipole-velocity method (155).

In a few special cases, the absolute configuration of compounds of the coupled-oscillator type (Sec. II-1), can be deduced from the
signs of the Cotton effect, when the exact geometric relationship of the chromophores in the
molecule and the direction of polarization of
the relevant electronic transitions are known.
This technique has been applied successfully to
the alkaloid calycanthine (34) and Tröger's base
(35), which have two aniline-type chromophores
(40,158).

As indicated previously (Sec. II-12), amino

acids containing an aromatic ring (e.g. phenyl-alanine, tyrosine, tryptophane, etc.) exhibit other Cotton effects besides the n–π* transition of the carboxyl group. If this is easily observed in tyrosine, in phenylalanine one observes only a weak Cotton effect around 260 nm. This is attributed to the local C_{2v} symmetry of the electrical and magnetical transition moment vectors in the benzene ring; these are perpendicular to each other in phenylalanine (42b). In tyrosine the mixing with the n–π* transitions destroys this orthogonality to some degree, whilst in phenylalanine only 3d- or σ-orbital can mix (42b,159).

a)   The aromatic quadrant rule:

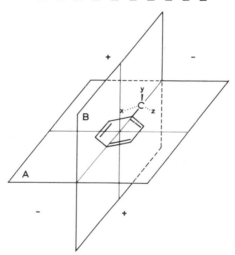

De Angelis, Wildman, Tetrahedron, **25**, 5099 (1969).

Fig. II-11.   The aromatic quadrant rule.

The CD properties of various rigid aromatic substances containing an asymmetric center adjacent to the aromatic ring have led to a quadrant rule, which allows to predict the absolute configuration when the structure is known (149).

This rule was developed on theoretical grounds for monosubstituted benzene compounds (44). As in the case of the carbonyl group, the benzene ring may be divided by planes through the p-orbitals (see Fig. II-11). Plane A passes through the six nodes of the π-orbitals of the aromatic ring, plane B is the symmetry plane (149).

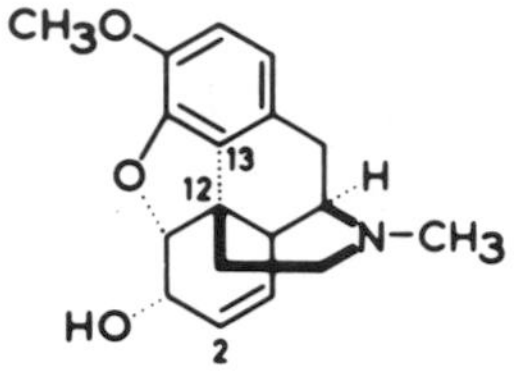

36 a

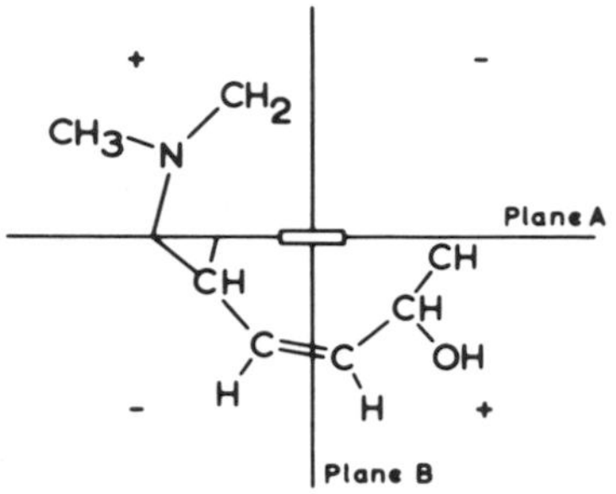

36 b

The aromatic quadrant rule, which has been tested with various aromatic alkaloids, is illustrated in the case of codeine (36a) (149). When the molecule is placed in quadrants, as shown on the projection (36b), the aromatic ring lies in plane A and is bisected by plane B. The methoxyl and epoxide groupings lie in plane A. If one looks at the molecule (36a) through C-2, C-12, and C-13, one gets the projection (36b) where groups in the upper-left and lower-right quadrants make positive contributions to the 240 nm Cotton effect. The substituents in the upper-right and lower-left quadrant give negative contributions. The signs are reversed when considering the 285 nm ($'A_{1g} \longrightarrow 'B_{2u}$) transition, because of the antipodal natures of "normal" aromatic ellipticities (149). In fact the Cotton effect of the 240 and 285 nm transitions in co-

deine (36a) is positive and negative, respectively, in agreement with the quadrant projection
(36b).

b)   The aromatic sector rule:

The examination of the chiroptical properties of tetrasubstituted aromatic substances,
belonging to the lycorine type of alkaloids, has
led to a sector rule which relates the sign and
magnitude of the Cotton effect to the spatial
orientation of atoms about the benzene chromophore (151).

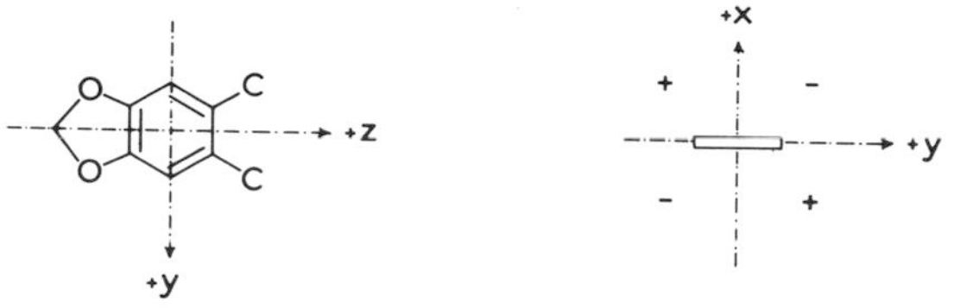

Kuriyama, Iwata, Moriyama, Kotera, Hamada, Mitsui, Takeda, J.C.S. (B), 46 (1967).

Fig. II-12. (I) Nodal and symmetry planes of
the 290 nm transition of the substituted benzene
chromophore and (II) octant projection.

Tetrasubstituted benzenes shown in Fig.
II-12 have C_{2v} local symmetry. The direction of
the electric dipole transition moment μe (equation [6]), for the 290 nm band, is along the z
two-fold axis of the chromophore. In compounds
of type shown in Fig. II-12, the scalar product
$\mu e.\mu m$ is not zero and the 290 nm transition is
optically active (151). If the benzene ring is
viewed along the $-z \longrightarrow +z$ axis, the contribution
of the group in each quadrant is as shown in Fig.
II-12.

The rule is illustrated in the case of β-
dihydrocaranine (37a) whose projection is shown

in (37b). The intense negative Cotton effect
exhibited by (37a) is attributed to the hydroxyl-
ated ring which falls in a negative sector (151).

37 a   37 b

        Besides the optical properties of more
flexible systems (160), various accounts have
appeared on the assignment of configuration to
representative members of the tetracyclin group
(161), as well as flavans, isoflavans, and related substances (148,162). In addition, many
detailed investigations have been published on
the chiroptical properties of lignans (148,163),
annulenes (164) and alkaloids (148), including
those of the yohimbane (165), keto-indole (166),
berberine (167), lycorine (151,168), quinoline
(148,169), and these of the Lythraceae (170), Nu-
phar (171), and Bulbocodium (172) families, as
well as various other aromatic chromophores (e.g.
quinones, tropones, pyrazoles, furans, quinoxa-
lines, pyridines, benzimidazoles, benzazocines,
spirobifluorenes etc.) (14,148,173,174). Finally, a theoretical treatment of the optical activity of bis-1,1'-spiroindanes has also appeared
(175).

c)   The benzoate sector rule:

        The strong Cotton effect of benzoates at-
tributed to $\pi-\pi^*$ intramolecular charge transfer
transition at ca. 225 nm permits to predict the
absolute configuration of a variety of cyclic
secondary hydroxyls. The benzoate sector rule,
shown in Fig. II-13, divides the space into four
sectors by symmetry planes A and B, and further

into eight sectors by two additional planes C and D perpendicular to A and passing through both oxygen atoms. The preferred conformation of the benzoyloxy group is assumed to be one in which it lies staggered between the carbinyl hydrogen and the smaller substituent (91).

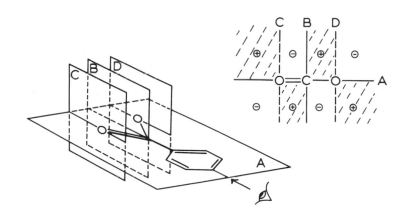

Harada, Ohashi, Nakanishi, J. A. C. S. **90**, 7349 (1968).

Fig. II-13.   The benzoate sector rule.

The benzoate is looked at from the para-position and the rotatory contributions of α,β and β,γ-bonds are considered. The sector rule states that bonds falling in the shaded and unshaded sectors in Fig. 11-13 make positive and negative contributions respectively to the 230 nm Cotton effect. The contributions of a double bond would be larger than that of a single bond because of the larger polarizability, and the sector which carries a β,γ-double bond, if any, will make the dominant contribution. Similarly, the sector carrying a γ,δ-double bond will define the sign of the Cotton effect when this is the unsaturation closest to the carbinyl carbon atom (91). Theoretical considerations (176) support the rule, which is illustrated in the case of p-substituted benzoates of cholesterol which exhibit positive Cotton effect ORD curves (a, from +115 to +207), in agreement with the rule (91,176).

The benzoate sector rule was applied to establish the absolute configuration of the antibiotic cervicarin (38a) (177). The CD curve of the p-chlorobenzoate (38b) shows two intense Cotton effects of opposite signs. The positive CD maximum at 242 nm indicates that the chirality between the long axes of the naphthalene and the p-chlorobenzoate chromophore is positive, i.e., the benzoate group has the β-configuration (177).

38 a   38 b

d)   The dibenzoate chirality rule:

In the case of cyclic α-glycol dibenzo-ates, the 230 nm absorption band is associated with two very strong Cotton effects of opposite signs at ca. 233 and 219 nm. This seems to indi-cate that both Cotton effects of dibenzoates are mainly due to a dipole interaction between elec-tric transition moments of the two benzoate chro-mophores. If the chiralities of dibenzoates are defined as being positive or negative, respec-tively, according to whether the rotation is in the sense of a right- or left-handed screw, then the sign of the first Cotton effect is in agree-ment with the chirality (91,178).

66

e)   The modified sector rules:

A sagacious examination of the various rules proposed for aromatic systems has led to modified sector rules for these chromophores (156). These rules are based on the concept of first, second and third sphere contributions (179). For the ^1L_b-band a sector rule has been proposed. The nodal planes pass through the C atoms of the benzene ring, whilst for the ^1L_a-band sector rule the nodal planes cross the mid-points of the benzene bonds. The plane of the aromatic ring was added as an additional nodal plane (179). A 6,7-dioxygenated tetralin presents a C_2-axis. A rotation around this axis does not change the signs of second and third sphere contributions. This requires a C_2-axis in the same direction for the corresponding sector rule, which means that in addition to the plane of the ring one other nodal plane should be added, which contains this C_2-axis and is perpendicular to the plane of the aromatic ring. The ^1L_a-sector rule has the correct symmetry for a tetralin and does not need any additional nodal plane (see schemes A and B in Fig. II-14). In benzene derivatives monosubstituted with a chiral group, a C_2-axis lies in the direction of the $C_{ar}-C^*$ bond, thus the fifth nodal plane has to be added in case of the ^1L_a-sector rule, but not for the ^1L_b-band (see schemes C and D in Fig. II-14) (156). Within small sectors containing the direction of projection, the signs of these modified sector rules are identical to these of previous rules (149,151).

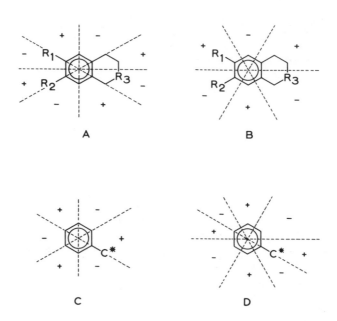

Snatzke, Ho, Tetrahedron, **27**, 3645 (1971).

Fig. II-14. Modified sector rules for third sphere contributions to the Cotton effects of the aromatic chromophore: R_1 and R_2 = H or OR', R_3 = CR_2'' or NR''. A: ^1L_b-band of tetralins and similar substances. B: ^1L_a-band of tetralins and similar compounds. C: ^1L_b-band of monosubstituted benzene chromophores. D: ^1L_a-band of monosubstituted benzenes.

f)   The styrene chirality rule:

          Examination of the geometry of the styrene chromophore with molecular models show that the chirality of the conjugated system in the Δ^6-aromatic steroids (39a) (right-handed helix; negative Cotton effect) is opposite to that in the $\Delta^{9(11)}$-compounds (39b) (left-handed helix; positive Cotton effect). Thus, a strong negative

Cotton effect associated with the 260-270 nm
transition indicates that the styrene chromophore is twisted in the form of a right-handed
helix.   Conversely, an intense positive Cotton
effect is indicative of a left-handed twist
(180).

39 a   **39 b**

The styrene chirality rule was also applied recently for the assignment of absolute
configuration to nafenopin, a 1-aryl-tetralin
(181), as well as to apo-compounds of the aryl-
naphthalene group (163).
      As in the case of skewed dienes (Sec. II-
4), substantial variations are sometimes observed
in the magnitude of the Cotton effect.   Moreover,
this rule should also be applied with caution to
new systems, mainly when unexpected electronic
and/or conformational factors are involved.

II-15. Episulfides, thiocarbonates and thiono-
carbonates.

The spectroscopic study of simple episulfides has indicated the presence of a low intensity UV maximum in the 260 nm region, which is
similar to the $n-\pi^*$ absorption of the carbonyl
chromophore.   The sign of the Cotton effect or
the rotational strength, or both parameters, can
be used for differentiating between the position
and/or configuration of the episulfide function
in steroid and triterpene molecules (72,182).
      As in carbonyl containing molecules, in
the case of the episulfide the experimental Cotton effect results only from the asymmetry in-

duced in the episulfide group by the vicinity.
Whereas the magnetic dipole moment of an n–π*
transition is directed along the internuclear
axis, it may be at right angles in an n–σ* transition, as in a sulfide. The shape of episulfide orbitals and the conformational factors responsible for the Cotton effect have been discussed (182) (see also Appendix, Sec. II-21).
    The sector rule proposed for the episul-
fide chromophore, explaining both the sign and
magnitude of the n–σ* Cotton effect, is illustrated in Fig. II-15 (72).
    In cyclic dithio- and trithiocarbonates,
if the plane formed by the two-ring heteroatoms
and the carbon atom of the thiocarbonyl group is
looked at from the thiocarbonyl sulfur atom
through its carbon atom, the sign of the n–π*
and π–π* Cotton effects will result from the
chirality of the chromophoric system as shown in
Table II-3 (72).

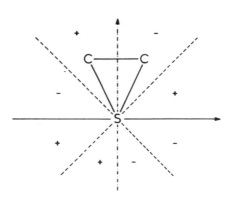

Kuriyama, Komeno, Takeda, Tetrahedron, **22**, 1039 (1966).

<u>Fig. II-15</u>.   The episulfide sector rule.

Table II-3

Sign of the Cotton Effects in Dithio- and Trithiocarbonates.

Chirality	Cotton effect	
	$n-\pi^*$ Transition	$\pi-\pi^*$ Transition
X —— S —— Y	Negative	Positive
X —— S —— Y	Positive	Negative

A study of model compounds of fixed conformations has shown a relationship between the
chirality of a cyclic thionocarbonate and the
sign of the Cotton effect associated with its
$n-\pi^*$ transition (183). The chirality of the
thionocarbonate ring may be defined as positive
or negative by viewing the ring from the sulfur
atom directly along the C=S bond (see Table II-
4).

Table II-4

Chirality and Cotton Effect of Thiocarbonate Ring in

C$_2$ Form (183).

Chirality	Cotton effect
	Positive
	Negative

II-16. Amines and derivatives.

Most molecules discussed above possess either an inherently dissymmetric chromophore or an inherently symmetric chromophore which is asymmetrically perturbed. However, some functional groups exhibit UV absorption bands below 220 or even 200 nm; such is the case of most aliphatic and alicyclic amines. Indeed, amines present a complex UV absorption pattern, usually at low wavelengths. UV of simple aliphatic amines in the vapor state show several transitions below 240 nm, two of which appear between 190 and 240 nm. In a study of the Cotton effects of tertiary amines, two optically active transitions have been observed, i.e., a weak absorption at ca. 220-230 nm and a more intense transition around 195-205 nm (184).

In the case of most aliphatic and alicyclic amines the stereochemistry cannot easily be ascertained from their chiroptical properties, since no Cotton effect appears in the spectral region commonly investigated with usual instruments. Then, one may refer to derivatives presenting more favorable spectroscopic properties. The ORD and CD data of a number of chromophoric derivatives of optically active amines and amino acids (see above) have been examined for their intrinsic spectroscopic interest, as well as to test their usefulness for the correlation of configuration. Among the most commonly used derivatives of the amino function are the isothiocyanate (87), the methylisothiocyanate (185), the nitrosoamines (186), nitrosoamides (186), nitrosites (187), alkylnitrites (188), Schiff bases (189,190) [such as N-benzylidene (191), N-isopropylidenes (192), N-salicylidenes (193)], phthalimides (194-196), maleyl (195,196), and itaconyl (196) derivatives, as well as N-phenylthioacetyl (197), N-thiobenzoyl (197,198), phenylthiohydantoins (199), sulphonamides (200), thionamides (15), etc. (see Table of chromophoric groups).

The Cotton effects associated with these chromophores and other derivatives of amines have been discussed in detail (14,15). Unfortunately, several of these derivatives are either difficult to prepare or lead to racemic mixtures; furthermore, some are unsuitable because they sometimes present undesirable optical properties. Among the various derivatives examined so far, the salicylidene chromophore, formed by condensation of salicylaldehyde with amines, is one of the most commonly used derivatives for the assignment of relative and/or absolute stereochemistry to optically active amines and amino acids (193). Usually amines with the (S)-configuration exhibit positive Cotton effect curves and (R)-derivatives, negative ORD and CD curves.

Other useful derivatives are the dimedone and dihydroresorcinol adducts. Usually, the dimedonyl derivatives of aliphatic and alicyclic amines having the (R)-configuration exhibit a positive Cotton effect in the 280 nm region. A negative Cotton effect is observed for compounds presenting the (S)-configuration (201). In addition, the intensity of the 280 nm Cotton effect varies with the type of amine, <u>e.g.</u> when the molecular amplitude of aliphatic amines is rather weak, in the case of saturated alicyclic amines, the intensity of the Cotton effect is a function of the conformational rigidity of the system. In ethylenic alicyclic amines and in aralkylamines, the intensity of the Cotton effects also depends on the proximity of the double bond or aromatic system to the vinylogous amide chromophore (201).

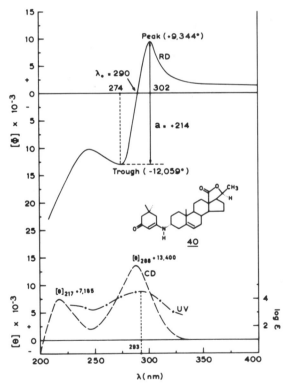

Fig. II-16. ORD, CD, and UV curves of N-(5,5-dimethyl-2-cyclohexen-1-on-3-yl)-gitingensine (<u>40</u>).

Fig. II-16 shows the ORD, CD, and UV curves of the N-(5,5-dimethyl-2-cyclohexen-1-on-3-yl) derivative of the steroidal alkaloid gitingensine (40). The dimedone derivative (40) contains a vinylogous amide chromophore absorbing at ca. 290 nm. The configuration at C-3 is (R) and the ORD curve is characterized by a positive Cotton effect, with a peak at 302 nm and a trough at 274 nm. The point λ_0 (290 nm) of rotation [Φ] = 0° where the curve inverts its sign, corresponds roughly to the wavelength of the CD maximum (288 nm) and of the UV band (293 nm) (Fig. II-16) (see Sec. I-3).

Compound (40) has also a lactone chromophore in its molecule. Since a positive Cotton effect is easily detected on the CD curve (around 217 nm), the (20S) absolute configuration could be established for the methyl, because isomeric (20R)-lactones show a negative Cotton effect in this spectral region (201). Worth noting is the strong negative background effect observed on the ORD curve in the low wavelengths region, which obliterates the lactone Cotton effect. Hence from the CD curve shown in Fig. II-16 the absolute configuration could be assigned to the carbon atoms C-3 and C-20 of the alkaloid derivative (40) (201).

Although the UV properties are very similar, the experimental ORD Cotton effect of dimedonyl derivatives can vary from a = 8, in the aliphatic series, to a = 960, in the aliphatic and alicyclic series, and to a = 1570 in the aromatic series (201). Thus, the intensity of a Cotton effect does not necessarily reflect the nature of the chromophore under investigation (inherently dissymmetric viz. inherently symmetric but asymmetrically perturbed).

In addition, the Cotton effects of dimedone and dihydroresorcinol condensation compounds of amino acids and some peptides have also been reported (201,202).

In the case of optically active aralkylamines, the Cotton effects of the aromatic transitions will sometimes give useful stereochemical information (42b,148,203). Very often, how-

ever, one is dealing with multiple Cotton effects ORD and CD curves. In addition, a change
in the nature of the substituent on the aromatic
ring, or in its position will affect the sign
and the intensity of the Cotton effects, sometimes rendering correlation of configuration difficult.

Fortunately, a quadrant sector rule has
been proposed for the 245-270 nm Cotton effects
of α- and β-phenylalkylamine hydrochlorides
(204). A previous rule, suggested on the basis
of the ORD data of a series of optically active
α-substituted phenylethanes and 1-substituted
indans, constitutes the first attempt to correlate the sign of the Cotton effects with the configuration of arylamines (205). The quadrant
sector rule, as applied to α-substituted phenylethanes and 1-substituted indanes is represented
in Fig. II-17 (204).

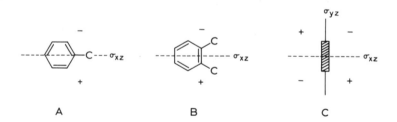

Smith, Willis, J. A. C. S., **93**, 2282 (1971).

Fig. II-17. The quadrant sector rule for aralkylamines: σ_{xz} and σ_{yz} are the symmetry planes
defined by the C_2 symmetry axis and by the plane
of the phenyl ring.

In A and B (Fig. II-17), the signs refer to the rotatory contributions of substituents or groups lying above the plane of the aromatic ring. For the groups below this plane the signs are reversed, as shown in C, viewed remotely from the ring substituents. Groups situated in the symmetry planes do not contribute to the rotatory perturbation (204).

The sign of the Cotton effects in the 245-270 nm region exhibited by various arylamine hydrochlorides can be predicted by this sector rule. This rule applies to an aromatic transition with the electric dipole transition moment perpendicular to the symmetry axis and in the ring plane (204).

II-17. Dithiocarbamates and dithiourethanes.

Besides the amino-derivatives listed in Sections II-12 and II-16, the N-nitrobenzoyl (206) and dithiocarbamate (199,207) chromophores are also used quite often for the determination of configuration of optically active amines and α-amino acids.

The 340 nm band of asymmetric dithiocarbamates and dithiourethanes is assigned to an n-π* transition, whilst the absorption at ca. 280 nm is attributed to a π-π* transition. A simple quadrant rule has been proposed (208) for the n-π* Cotton effect of dithiocarbamates. This rule illustrated in Fig. II-18, allows to predict the sign of the Cotton effects. Substituents falling in the upper-right and lower-left quadrants make a positive contribution, whereas substituents in upper-left and lower-right quadrants make negative contributions to the Cotton effect.

Although the Cotton effect associated with the n-π* transition of the NCS_2 chromophore is rather weak, the quadrant rule for dithiocarbamates has been successfully applied to various aliphatic and alicyclic amino-derivatives (208).

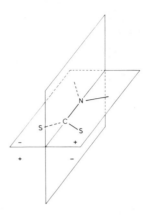

Ripperger, Tetrahedron, <u>25</u>, 725 (1969)

Fig. II-18. The quadrant rule for the dithiocarbamate chromophore.

II-18. <u>Azides</u>.

Alkyl azides show a rather weak transition around 285 nm attributed to the promotion of an electron from a nonbonding $2p_y$ orbital situated mainly on the nitrogen atom N_1 concerned with bonding to the alkyl group, to an antibonding π_x^* orbital associated principally with $2p_x$ atomic orbitals from the remaining two nitrogen atoms (N_2 and N_3).

An octant rule for the azide chromophore has been proposed (209). As in the case of the saturated ketone, only two of the surfaces specifying the octants are well defined in terms of symmetry. In order to determine the sign associated with a particular octant, one has to look at the chromophore along the N_3-N_2-N_1 axis from N_3 towards N_1 the bond specifying the lone pair of electrons on N_1 lying in a vertical plane, as indicated in Fig. II-19. The signs of the azide octants are the same as those of the carbonyl octants (209).

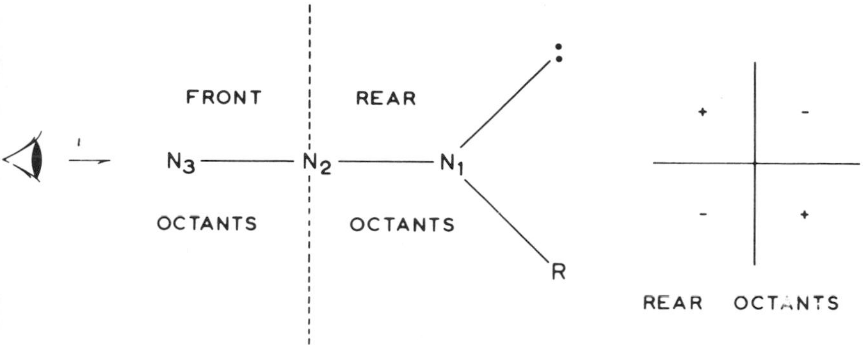

Djerassi, Moscowitz, Ponsold, Steiner, J.A.C.S, **89**, 347 (1967).

<u>Fig. II-19</u>. The octant rule for the azide chromophore.

The rule is illustrated in the case of 7α-azido cholesterol acetate (<u>41</u>). Since most of the tetracyclic system falls in the upper-right octant, compound (<u>41</u>) presents a negative molecular ellipticity ($[\theta]_{290}$ -2040) (209).

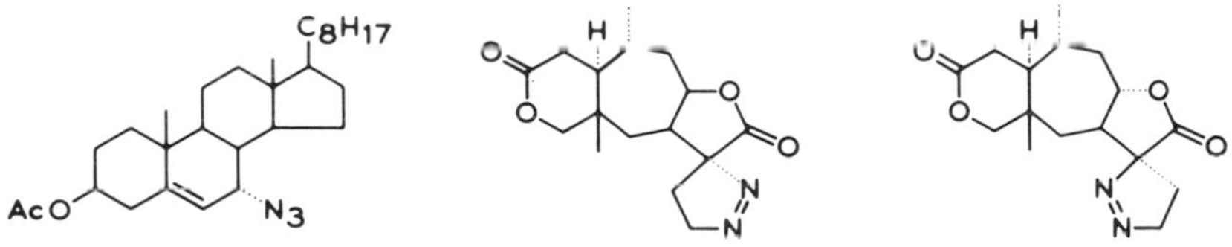

The azide octant rule can be applied to some azido-sugars, but both the conformation of the ring-system as well as the configuration of the substituents should be taken into consideration (210).

II-19. <u>Azomethines, nitrosoamines, N-chloro-amines, nitro-, nitryloxy-derivatives, aziridines, pyrazolines.</u>

Several rules predicting the sign of the

Cotton effect of cyclic azomethines (211), nitro-soamines, nitro-derivatives (186,212), as well as N-chloroamines (213) are now available.

The C=N chromophore of azomethines shows a weak absorption around 250 nm, which becomes optically active in a dissymmetric surrounding. A rule, based on numerous examples, states that cyclic azomethines of conformation (V) exhibit a positive Cotton effect, whereas a negative Cotton effect is associated with conformation (VI) (211).

V   VI

The $n_N- \pi_3^*$ transition of N-nitroso-derivatives of optically active amines appears in the 370 nm region and exhibits a Cotton effect, function of the stereochemistry in its vicinity. A sector rule illustrated in Fig. II-18 has been proposed for this chromophore (186,212).

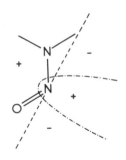

Snatzke, Ripperger, Horstman, Schreiber, Tetrahedron, **22**, 3103 (1966)

Fig. II-20. The sector rule for the N-nitroso-chromophore.

N-chloroamines and N-chloroamino-ketals exhibit a weak absorption band between 250 and 280 nm, and a correlation between the stereochemistry in the vicinity of the chromophore and the sign of the Cotton effect has been established (213). It should be mentioned, however, that the N-chlor- and N-nitrosamine rule seems to present some exceptions (214).

A sector rule, shown in Fig. II-21, has been derived for the nitro-chromophore from the CD data obtained on numerous compounds (7,212, 215).

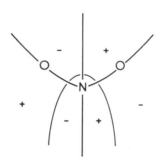

Snatzke, J. C. S., 5002 (1965).

Fig. II-21. The sector rule for the nitro-chromophore.

The spiro-pyrazoline derivative of monoterpenes, sesquiterpene lactones, and homo-conjugated dienes, as well as of some steroids has been prepared (216). The azo group of this heterocycle is optically active in an asymmetric vicinity. Its Cotton effect, which appears at ca. 330 nm, is enhanced by the presence of a carbonyl in the vicinity (216).

The pyrazoline derivative of floribundin and vermeerin proved to be a convenient chromophore for the assignment of configuration of the methylene-γ-lactone grouping in these isomeric sesquiterpene di-lactones. Indeed, the pyrazoline of floribundin (42) exhibits a positive molecular ellipticity ($[\theta]_{319}$ +11,800), whilst the pyrazoline of vermeerin (43) shows a negative CD

curve ($[\theta]_{324}$ -10,000). These Cotton effects
indicate that addition of diazomethane to the
methylene group takes place from the α face and
β face, respectively, thus supporting the cis
and trans configuration of the γ-lactone in these
sesquiterpenes (216).

In nitryloxy-steroids, three weak Cotton
effects are detected in the 270, 230, and 210 nm
region. These CD bands can be used for the location of hydroxyl groupings as well as for stereochemical assignments (217).

An asymmetrical center in 2-alkylaziridine
determines the formation of a stable asymmetric
nitrogen atom in stereoselective N-halogenation
reactions. The ORD properties of some halogenated aziridines have been reported (218).

II-20. The thiocyanate chromophore.

The optical properties of the isothio-
cyanato (87) and methylisothiocyanato (185) derivatives of some amino alcohols, amino acids,
and peptides have been reported. In addition,
ORD and CD studies of a number of steroidal thiocyanates have demonstrated that the 250 nm transition is optically active (219). It has been
assumed that this transition is qualitatively
similar to the n-π* transition of azides so that
an octant rule, illustrated in Fig. II-22, has
been proposed for this chromophore.

The optical activity associated with the
azide chromophore (209), classified as inherently
symmetric, suggests that similar arguments might
apply to the iso-electric thiocyanate chromophore
(-S-C≡N). Hence, any optical activity associated
with these groups follows as a consequence of
their being located in a dissymmetric molecular
environment. Accordingly, the sign and the magnitude of their Cotton effect will depend on the
nature and location of the atoms in the vicinity
of the chromophore. The thiocyanate transition,
at ca. 245 nm, may be attributed to the promotion
of an electron from a nonbonding $3p_y$-orbital sit-

uated mainly on sulfur to an antibonding π^*-orbital determined largely by the carbon and nitrogen $2p_x$-atomic orbitals (219).

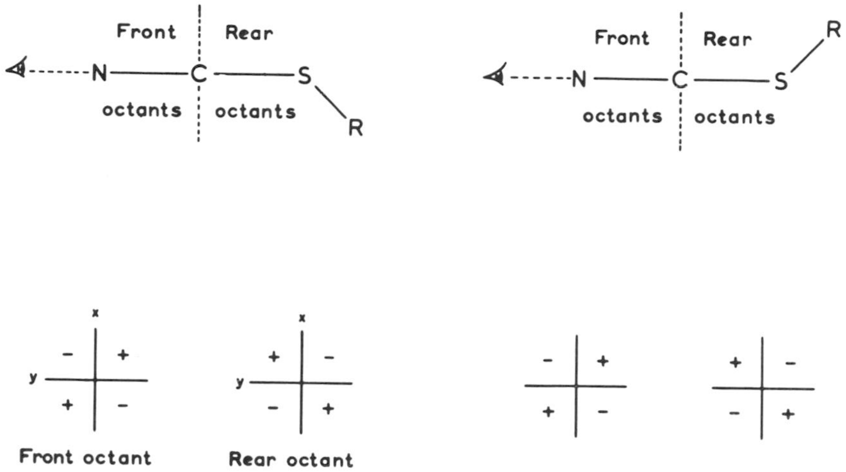

Djerassi, Lightner, Schooley, Takeda, Komeno, Kuriyama,

Tetrahedron, **24**, 6913 (1968).

Fig. II-22. The octant rule for the thiocyanate chromophore.

　　　　Looking along the axis from nitrogen through carbon to sulfur (see Fig. II-22), the symmetry planes are: a) xz-plane containing the S, C, and N atoms and the carbon of group R attached to sulfur; b) the yz-plane, which is orthogonal to the xz-plane, and contains the S, C, and N atoms; c) a so far poorly defined surface approximated by a third plane (xy), orthogonal to the other planes and passing through the carbon atom of the S-C≡N grouping (219).
　　　　As in the case of azide, the rotational strength of the thiocyanate chromophore, is weaker than that of the carbonyl group. The CD data of various thiosteroids have been obtained, and the potential utility of the new octant rule has been demonstrated by analyzing the rotameric contributions of various steroidal thiocyanates.

Temperature-dependent CD curves of such derivatives have also been obtained in order to study the effect of free rotation (219).

II-21. Other sulfur derivatives, disulfides, sulfoxides, phosphorus containing chromophores, etc.

Besides the chromophores mentioned above, several other sulfur containing functional groups have been examined by the ORD and CD techniques. Among the functions investigated, one should mention the xanthates (220,221), dithiocarboxy groups (208), dithiocarbamates (199,207,221), thionocarbalkoxy derivatives (159,199), thiohydantoines (15,199), acylthioureas (223), sulfides (224), dithianes (225), dithiolans (226), thiones (227), thioethers (228), sulfoxides and related compounds (229).

The optical properties of active organic sulfites (230) and alkylsulfinyl-steroids (231) have been reported. Furthermore, the influence of ethylene-acetal, monothioacetal, and dithioacetal functions on the Cotton effect associated with a vicinal ketone has been discussed (232).

The ORD curves of sulfimides and sulfoximides have been obtained. A correlation has been established between the Cotton effects and the configuration of these functional groups (233). The CD spectrum of sulfenamides demonstrates that this chromophore presents a number of optically active transitions in the 195-290 nm region (234).

The study of the chiroptical properties of various phosphine oxides and phosphine sulfides has led to a direct configurational correlation of sulfoxides and phosphine oxides by intersystem matching of the Cotton effects (235). The similarity in the dichroism of the two systems suggests the possibility of a displacement rule embracing sulfoxides and phosphine oxides. At a wavelength λ, removed from the center of the optically active transitions, the molecular rotation $[\Phi]$ is proportional to the sum over all transitions $\lambda_i^2 R_i / (\lambda^2 - \lambda_i^2)$, where λ_i and R_i are the position of the band center and the rotational strength of the ith transition respectively (235).

Each pair of compounds is known, from external evidence, to have the same absolute configuration and to differ only in the replacement of a $S=O$ group by a $CH_3-P=O$ group, and by one methyl at a remote position in one aromatic ring (44) and (45). The CD curves of the sulfoxides correspond closely in sign and shape to those of the phosphine oxides. This is a dramatic confirmation of the independently-assigned absolute configurations (235).

44   45

Various studies have been devoted to the examination of the chiroptical properties of other phosphorus containing optically active substances (e.g. phenylphosphinates, biphenylone-phosphorus ions, phenylphosphine oxide, etc.) (235,236).

The optical properties of asymmetric thiepan-2-ones and poly(thiol esters) have also been investigated (237). Two Cotton effects centered around 298 nm (n-π* transition) and 234 nm (π-π* band) are associated with the thiolactone chromophore.

The disulfide chromophore (-S-S-) is of particular importance in chemistry and biochemistry. This functional group exhibits various UV bands which are optically active (182,225,238). Usually, the first UV transition in open-chain disulfides lacks inherent optical activity, whereas a strong optical activity is observed in cyclic

disulfides (54). Six-membered ring systems with
the disulfide chromophore twisted in the sense
of a left-handed helix show an intense negative
Cotton effect around 280-290 nm, attributed to
the inherently dissymmetrical nature of the chromophore. A second Cotton effect of opposite
sign, reduced magnitude, and more sensitive to
minor perturbations appears at ca. 240 nm (54,
238). For instance, three optically active transitions, attributed to the disulfide chromophore,
are observed in the metabolite acetylaranotin
(46) at 345, 310, and 268 nm. The chemical
transformation of (46), closely related to the
antibiotic gliotoxin (47), yields the diol (48).
The CD of this diol (48) shows only three Cotton
effects (222,210 and below 200 nm) below 230 nm
corresponding to the cyclic diketopiperazine
chromophore (133,239) (Sec. IV-1), thus indicating that in acetylaranotin (46) the optically
active transitions at higher wavelengths are due
to the disulfide grouping (238).

46   **47**   **48**

II-22. Ethers, ozonides, nitrones, nitroxides,
imines, C-nitroso compounds, polyenes,
etc.

The optical properties of some aliphatic
and cyclic ethers (tetrahydrofuran, tetrahydro-
pyran) and their complexes (240), as well as
thioethers (228) have been reported. ORD curves
of ozonides have been obtained (241).
A number of nitroxides has been prepared.
Among them camphenyl t-butyl nitroxide has been
shown to be a stable, optically active, free rad-
ical, of which the CD has been studied (242).
At least four transitions have been found

to be associated with the nitrone chromophore
($\overset{+}{>}$C=N-$\overset{-}{O}$); i.e., a weak n-π^* band at ca. 295 nm,
a strong π-π^* transition around 230-250 nm, an
n-σ^* band at ca. 207 nm, and a fourth transition
presumably of π-π^* type. In an asymmetric vicinity, these transitions become optically active (243). Photochemical treatment of nitrones
affords oxazirans. The oxaziran group

($>$C$\overset{O}{\diagup\diagdown}$N —) is also an optically active chromophore, which presents at least two Cotton ef-
fects (i.e., around 225 nm and 195 nm) (244).
The chiroptical properties of aliphatic
C-nitroso compounds which present several optically active transitions have been reported (245).
In addition, studies of the azoxy chromophore
(246), imines (76,248), and ureides (228), as
well as of 3-methylpyrrolidin-2-one (249) and of
the dithiocarbethoxy derivative of an antibiotic
(250) have also appeared. The CD properties of
the 3-cephem chromophore, the basic skeleton of
the cephalosphorin antibiotics, are typified by
bands of opposite signs at ca. 220-260 nm (251).
Conjugated polyenes belonging to the
carotenoid family display several Cotton effects
between 200 and 400 nm (252). The sign and intensity of these Cotton effects reflect the stereochemistry at the chiral end-groups. ORD and
CD data have allowed to correlate compounds belonging to different series and to assign the
absolute configuration to various substances per-
taining to this class of poly-olefins. For example, the chirality of carotenes, α-cryptoxanthin,
crocoxanthin, and xanthophyll has been established. Furthermore, ORD and CD have shown the
chirality at C-6 to be the same in natural (+)-
α-carotene, (+)- δ-carotene, and ε-carotene (252).
Finally, several studies have been devoted to the optical properties of some compounds
in which the asymmetric center is different from
carbon, sulfur, phosphorus, or nitrogen (e.g. Si,
Ge, Se, Te, etc.) (14,253).

References

63. A.K. Bose, M.S. Manhas, R.C. Cambie, and L.N. Mander, J. Amer. Chem. Soc., 84, 3201 (1962); Tetrahedron, 20, 409 (1964); C. Djerassi, H. Wolf, and E. Bunnenberg, J. Amer. Chem. Soc., 85, 324 (1963); P.A. Hart and M.P. Tripp, Chem. Comm., 174 (1969); S. Sarel, Y. Shalon, Y. Yanuka, Tetrahedron Letters, 957, 961 (1969); M. Ribi and C.H. Eugster, Helv. Chim. Acta, 52, 1732 (1969).

64. B.A. Chaudri, D.G. Goodwin, H.R. Hudson, L. Bartlett, and P.M. Scopes, J. Chem. Soc. (C), 1329 (1970); R.C. Cookson and J.M. Coxon, J. Chem. Soc. (C), 1466 (1971).

65. A.W. Burgstahler, R.C. Barkhurst, and J.A. Gawronski, in Modern Methods of Steroid Analysis, E. Heftmann (edit.), Academic Press, Inc., New York, in press.

66. A. Yogev and Y. Mazur, Chem. Comm., 552 (1965); Tetrahedron, 22, 1317 (1966); A. Yogev, D. Amar, and Y. Mazur, Chem. Comm., 339 (1967).

67. A.I. Scott and A.D. Wrixon, Chem. Comm., 1182 (1969); 43 (1970); Tetrahedron, 26, 3695 (1970); D.P. Della Casa de Macano, T.G. Halsall, A.I. Scott, and A.D. Wrixon, Chem. Comm., 582 (1970); Tetrahedron, 27, 4787 (1971).

68. M. Fétizon and I. Hanna, Chem. Comm., 462 (1970); I. Hanna, Ph.D. Thesis, University of Paris (1970).

69. M. Fétizon, I. Hanna, A.I. Scott, A.D. Wrixon, and T.K. Devon, Chem. Comm., 545 (1971); J. Gawronski and M.A. Kielczewski, Tetrahedron Letters, 2493 (1971); A.I. Scott and A.D. Wrixon, Tetrahedron, in press.

70. M. Legrand and R. Viennet, Compt. rend., 262, 1290 (1966); R. Rossi, L. Lardicci, and G. Ingrosso, Tetrahedron, 26, 4067 (1970); R. Rossi and P. Diversi, Tetrahedron, 26, 5033 (1970).

71. E. Bunnenberg and C. Djerassi, J. Amer. Chem. Soc., 82, 5953 (1960).

72. C. Djerassi, H. Wolf, D.A. Lightner, E. Bunnenberg, K. Takeda, T. Komeno, and K. Kuriyama, Tetrahedron, 19, 1547 (1963); D.A. Lightner and C. Djerassi, Tetrahedron, 21, 583 (1965); D.A. Lightner, C. Djerassi, K. Takeda, K. Kuriyama, and T. Komeno, Tetrahedron, 21, 1581 (1965); K. Kuriyama, T. Komeno, and K. Takeda, Tetrahedron, 22, 1039 (1966).

73. A.H. Haines and C.S.P. Yenkins, Chem. Comm., 350 (1969).

74. E. Premuzic and A.I. Scott, Chem. Comm., 1078 (1967); A.D. Wrixon, E. Premuzic, and A.I. Scott, Chem. Comm., 639 (1968).

75. A.I. Scott and A.D. Wrixon, Chem. Comm., 1184 (1969); Tetrahedron, 27, 2339 (1971).

76. S.F. Mason and G.W. Vane, Chem. Comm., 540 (1965).

77. A. Moscowitz, E. Charney, U. Weiss, and H. Ziffer, J. Amer. Chem. Soc., 83, 4661 (1961); U. Weiss, H. Ziffer, and E. Charney, Tetrahedron, 21, 3105 (1965); H. Ziffer, U. Weiss, G.R. Narayanan, and R.V. Pachapurkar, J. Org. Chem., 31, 2691 (1966); H.J.C. Jacobs and E. Havinga, Rec. Trav. Chim., 84, 932 (1965).

78. P. Crabbé and A. Guzman, Third Natural Products Symposium, Mona (Jamaica), January 1970, Abstracts of papers, p. 10; P. Crabbe and G. Guzmán, Chem. and Ind., 851 (1971).

79. P. Crabbé, Proc. Natl. Acad. Sci. U.S., 66, 232 (1970).

80a. S. Bory and C.R. Engel, Bull. Soc. Chim. France, 3043 (1970); C.R. Engel and L. Ruest, Canad. J. Chem., 48, 3136 (1970); J. Lessard, L. Ruest, and Ch. Engel, in press.

80b. A.F. Beecham, A. McL. Mathieson, S.R. Johns, J.A. Lamberton, A.A. Sioumis, T.J. Batterham and I.G. Young, Tetrahedron, 27, 3725 (1971).

80c. P. Crabbé in Modern Methods of Steroid Analysis, E. Heftmann (edit.), Academic Press, Inc., New York, in press.

81. A.W. Burgstahler and R.C. Barkhurst, J. Amer. Chem. Soc., 92, 7601 (1970); A.W. Burgstahler, J. Gawronski, T.F. Niemann, and B.A. Feinberg, Chem. Comm., 121 (1971).

82. E. Charney, H. Ziffer, and U. Weiss, Tetrahedron, 21, 3121 (1965).

83. K. Mislow, Ann. N.Y. Acad. Sci., 93, 459 (1962); D.J. Sandman and K. Mislow, J. Amer. Chem. Soc., 91, 645 (1969); B. Bosnich, A. De Renzi, G. Paiaro, J. Himmelreich, and G. Snatzke, Inorg. Chim. Acta, 3, 175 (1969).

84. G. Lowe, Chem. Comm., 411 (1965); J.H. Brewster, Topic in Stereochemistry, N.L. Allinger and E.L. Eliel (edit.), vol. 2, John Wiley, New York, (1967).

85. P. Crabbé, E. Velarde, H.W. Anderson, S.D. Clark, W.R. Moore, A.F. Drake, and S.F. Mason, Chem. Comm., 1261 (1971).

86. P. Crabbé, E. Velarde, A.F. Drake, and S.F. Mason, in press.

87. B. Halpern, W. Patton, and P. Crabbé, J. Chem. Soc. (B) 1143 (1969).

88. S.T.K. Bukhari, R.D. Guthrie, A.I. Scott, and A.D. Wrixon, Chem. Comm., 1580 (1968); Tetrahedron, 26, 3653 (1970).

89. See ref. 14; also: S. Inouye, T. Tsuruoka, and T. Niida, J. Antibiotics, 19, 288 (1966); S. Inouye, Chem. Pharm. Bull. Japan, 15, 1609 (1967); R.C. Schulz, R. Wolf, and H. Mayerhöfer, Kolloid Zeitsch. and Zeitsch. Polym., 227, 65 (1968); K. Heyns, K.W. Pflughaupt, and H. Paulsen, Chem. Ber., 101, 2800 (1968); W.S. Chilton, J. Org. Chem., 33, 4459 (1968); T. Sticzay, C. Peciar, and S. Bauer, Tetrahedron Letters, 2407 (1968); M. Maeda, T. Kinoshita, and A. Tsuji, Tetrahedron Letters, 3407 (1968); I. Listowsky and S. England, Biochem. Biophys. Res. Comm., 30, 329 (1968); G.G. Lyle and M.J. Piazza, J. Org. Chem., 33, 2478 (1968); S. Inouye, T. Tsuruoka, T. Ito, and T. Niida, Tetrahedron, 24, 2125 (1968); H. Iwamura and T. Hashizume, J. Org. Chem., 33, 1796 (1968); H. Paulsen, J. Brüning, and K. Heyns, Chem. Ber., 102, 459 (1969); H. Paulsen, K. Propp,

and J. Brüning, Chem. Ber., 102, 469 (1969);
F. Cramer, G. Mackensen, and K. Sensse,
Chem. Ber., 102, 494 (1969); K. Sensse and
F. Cramer, Chem. Ber., 102, 509 (1969); R.J.
Ferrier, N. Prasad, and G.H. Sankey, J.
Chem. Soc. (C), 587 (1969); T. Sticzay, C.
Peciar, and S. Bauer, Tetrahedron, 25, 3521
(1969); H. Paulsen and F. Leupold, Chem.
Ber., 102, 2804, 2822 (1969); L. Mester, H.
El Khadem, and G. Vass, Tetrahedron Letters,
4135 (1969); D.K. Fukushima and M. Matsui,
Steroids, 14, 649 (1969), and references
therein; S. Beychok and G. Ashwell, Carbohyd.
Res., 17, 19 (1971).

90. L. Velluz and M. Legrand, Compt. rend., 263,
1429 (1966); W. Voelter, E. Bayer, R.
Records, E. Bunnenberg, and C. Djerassi,
Ann. Chem., 718, 238 (1968); W. Voelter, G.
Kuhfittig, G. Schneider, and E. Bayer, Ann.
Chem., 734, 126 (1970); Chem. Ber., 104,
1234 (1971).

91. N. Harada, M. Ohashi, and K. Nakanishi, J.
Amer. Chem. Soc., 90, 7349 (1968); N. Harada,
H. Sato, and K. Nakanishi, Chem. Comm., 1691
(1970).

92. K. Nakanishi and J. Dillon, J. Amer. Chem.
Soc., 93, 4058 (1971); Chem. Comm., 1235 (1971).

93. C. Faget, J.M. Conia, and E.H. Eschinazi,
Compt. rend., 258, 600 (1964); J.M. Conia
and J. Gore, Bull. Soc. Chim. France, 1968
(1964); J. Gore, C. Djerassi, and J.M. Conia,
Bull. Soc. Chim. France, 950 (1967); W.F.
Erman, R.S. Treptow, P. Bakuzis, and E.
Wenkert, J. Amer. Chem. Soc., 93, 657 (1971).

94. C. Ouannes, C. Ouannes, and J. Jacques,
Compt. rend., 257, 2118 (1963); D. Varech,
C. Ouannes, and J. Jacques, Bull. Soc. Chim.
France, 1662 (1965); C. Ouannes and J.
Jacques, Bull. Soc. Chim. France, 3601, 3611
(1965); C. Djerassi, R. Records, C. Ouannes,
and J. Jacques, Bull. Soc. Chim. France,
2378 (1966); S. Feinleib and F.A. Bovey,
Chem. Comm., 978 (1968); R. Filler and C.S.
Wang, Chem. Comm., 287 (1968); O. Schnepp,
E.F. Pearson, and E. Sharman, Chem. Comm.,

545 (1970); M.J. Brienne, A. Heymes, J. Jacques, G. Snatzke, W. Klyne, and S.R. Wallis, J. Chem. Soc. (C), 423 (1970); F.S. Richardson, D.D. Shillady, J.E. Bloor, J. Phys. Chem., 75, 2466 (1971).

95. C. Djerassi and G.W. Krakower, J. Amer. Chem. Soc., 81, 237 (1959); T. Sato, H. Minato, M. Shiro, and H. Koyama, Chem. Comm., 363 (1966); L. Kohout and J. Fajkoš, Coll. Czechosl. Chem. Comm., 34, 2439 (1969); J.B. Jones and J.M. Zander, Canad. J. Chem., 47, 3501 (1969); J. Levisalles and G. Teutsch, Bull. Soc. Chim. France, 263 (1971).

96. J.Y. Carsim and J.T. Yang, Biochem., 8, 1947 (1969); D.F. De Tar, Anal. Chem., 41, 1406 (1969); W.C. Krueger and L.M. Pschigoda, Anal. Chem., 43, 675 (1971).

97. P. Crabbé, L.H. Zalkow, and N.N. Girotra, J. Org. Chem., 30, 1678 (1965); see also ref. 14.

98. J. Padilla, J. Romo, F. Walls, and P. Crabbé, Rev. Soc. Quím. Méx., 11, 7 (1967); see also ref. 14.

99. J.S.E. Holker, W.R. Jones, M.G.R. Leeming, G.M. Holder, and W.B. Whalley, Chem. Comm., 90 (1967); J. Hudec, Chem. Comm., 539 (1967); G. Snatzke and G. Eckhardt, Tetrahedron, 24, 4543 (1968); 26, 1143 (1970); G. Snatzke, B. Ehrig, and H. Klein, Tetrahedron, 25, 5601 (1969); M.E. Herr, R.A. Johnson, W.C. Krueger, H.C. Murray, and L.M. Pschigoda, J. Org. Chem., 35, 3607 (1970); L. Bartlett, D.N. Kirk, W. Klyne, S.R. Wallis, H. Erdtman, and S. Thorén, J. Chem. Soc. (C), 2678 (1970); C. Coulombeau and A. Rassat, Bull. Soc. Chim. France, 516 (1971); J. Hudec, Chem. Comm., 829 (1970); M.T. Hughes and J. Hudec, Chem. Comm., 805 (1971); G.P. Powell and J. Hudec, Chem. Comm., 806 (1971).

100. M. Legrand, R. Viennet, and J. Caumartin, Compt. rend., 253, 2378 (1961); C. Djerassi, W. Klyne, T. Norin, G. Ohloff, and E. Klein, Tetrahedron, 21, 163 (1965); T.M. Feeley and M.K. Hargreaves, J. Chem. Soc. (C), 1745 (1970).

101. P. Leriverend and J.M. Conia, Bull. Soc.
     Chim. France, 121 (1966).
102. H.C. Brown and A. Suzuki, J. Amer. Chem.
     Soc., 89, 1933 (1967); S.B. Laing and P.J.
     Sykes, J. Chem. Soc. (C), 937 (1968).
103. K. Kuriyama, H. Tada, Y.K. Sawa, S. Itô,
     and I. Itoh, Tetrahedron Letters, 2539
     (1968); W. Reusch and P. Mattison, Tetra-
     hedron, 24, 4933 (1968); F.K. Butcher, R.A.
     Coombs, and M.T. Davies, Tetrahedron, 24,
     4041 (1968).
104. J.R. Bull and P.R. Enslin, Tetrahedron, 26,
     1525 (1970).
105. D.F. Morrow, M.E. Butler, and E.C.Y. Huang,
     J. Org. Chem., 30, 579 (1965); J. Hudec,
     Chem. Comm., 829 (1970); A.H. Beckett, A.Q.
     Khokhar, G.P. Powell, and J. Hudec, Chem.
     Comm., 326 (1971).
106. D.A. Lightner and W.A. Beavers, J. Amer.
     Chem. Soc., 93, 2677 (1971).
107. P. Crabbé, A. Cruz, and J. Iriarte, Chem.
     and Ind., 1522 (1967); Canad. J. Chem., 46,
     349 (1968).
108. W.B. Whalley, Chem. and Ind., 1024 (1962);
     R.E. Ballard, S.F. Mason, and G.W. Vane,
     Disc. Faraday Soc., 35, 43 (1963); G.
     Snatzke, Tetrahedron, 21, 413, 421, 439
     (1965).
109. A. Moscowitz, Communication at the NATO
     Summer School on ORD and CD, Bonn, September
     1965; K. Kuriyama, M. Moriyama, T. Iwata,
     and K. Tori, Tetrahedron Letters, 1661
     (1968); R. Bucourt, D. Hainaut, J.C. Gasc,
     and G. Nominé, Tetrahedron Letters, 5093
     (1968).
110. S. Imai, E. Murata, S. Fujioka, T. Matsuoka,
     M. Koreeda, and K. Nakanishi, J. Amer.
     Chem. Soc., 92, 7510 (1970).
111. C. Djerassi, R. Records, E. Bunnenberg, K.
     Mislow, and A. Moscowitz, J. Amer. Chem.
     Soc., 84, 870 (1962).
112. H. Ziffer and C.H. Robinson, Tetrahedron,
     24, 5803 (1968).
113a. L. Velluz, M. Legrand, and R. Viennet,
     Compt. rend., 261, 1687 (1965).

113b. R.N. Totty and J. Hudec, Chem. Comm., 785 (1971).

114. P. Crabbé, R. Grezemkovsky, and L.H. Knox, Bull. Soc. Chim. France, 789 (1968); P. Crabbé, P. Anderson, and E. Velarde, J. Amer. Chem. Soc., 90, 2998 (1968); P. Anderson, P. Crabbé, A.D. Cross, J.H. Fried, L.H. Knox, J. Murphy, and E. Velarde, J. Amer. Chem. Soc., 90, 3888 (1968); P. Crabbé, H. Carpio, and E. Velarde, Chem. Comm., 1028 (1971).

115. Z. Kis, A. Closse, H.P. Sigg, L. Hruban, and G. Snatzke, Helv. Chim. Acta, 53, 1577 (1970).

116. E. Bunnenberg, C. Djerassi, K. Mislow, and A. Moscowitz, J. Amer. Chem. Soc., 84, 2823, 5003 (1962).

117. P. Crabbé, A. Cruz, and J. Iriarte, Photochem. and Photobiol., 7, 829 (1968); P. Sunder-Plassman, P.H. Nelson, P.H. Boyle, A. Cruz, J. Iriarte, P. Crabbé, J.A. Zderic, J.A. Edwards, and J.H. Fried, J. Org. Chem., 34, 3779 (1969).

118. P. Crabbé, Tetrahedron, 20, 1211 (1964); P. Crabbé and A. Bowers, J. Org. Chem., 32, 2921 (1967); R.C. Cookson and J. Hudec, J. Chem. Soc., 429 (1962).

119. H.T. Thomas and K. Mislow, J. Amer. Chem. Soc., 92, 6292 (1970).

120. C. Djerassi and W. Klyne, J. Chem. Soc., 2390 (1963); T.D. Bouman and A. Moscowitz, J. Chem. Phys., 48, 3115 (1968).

121. J.P. Jennings, W. Klyne, and P.M. Scopes, J. Chem. Soc., 294, 7211, 7229 (1965); W. Klyne, P.M. Scopes, and A. Williams, J. Chem. Soc., 7237 (1965); W. Klyne, Proc. Roy. Soc., A, 297, 66 (1967); G. Gottarelli, W. Klyne, and P.M. Scopes, J. Chem. Soc (C), 1366 (1967); G. Gottarelli and P.M. Scopes, J. Chem. Soc. (C), 1370 (1967); J.D. Renwick and P.M. Scopes, J. Chem. Soc. (C), 1949 (1968); W. Klyne and P.M. Scopes, Il Farmaco, 24, 123 (1969); W.P. Mose and P.M. Scopes, J. Chem. Soc. (C), 2417 (1970).

122. A. Fredga, J.P. Jennings, W. Klyne, P.M.
      Scopes, B. Sjöberg, and S. Sjöberg, J.
      Chem. Soc., 3928 (1965); I.P. Dirkx and F.
      L.J. Sixma, Rec. Trav. Chim., 83, 522
      (1964); J. Cymerman Craig and S.K. Roy,
      Tetrahedron, 21, 1847 (1965); J. Cymerman
      Craig, D.P.G. Hamon, K.K. Purushothaman,
      S.K. Roy, and H.E.M. Lands, Tetrahedron,
      22, 175 (1966); Y. Inouye, S. Sawada, M.
      Ohno, and H.M. Walborsky, Tetrahedron, 23,
      3237 (1967); L. Verbit and Y. Inouye, J.
      Amer. Chem. Soc., 89, 5717 (1967); W.
      Klyne, P.M. Scopes, R.C. Sheppard, and S.
      Turner, J. Chem. Soc. (C), 1954 (1968); T.
      G. Waddell, W. Stöcklin, and T.A. Geissman,
      Tetrahedron Letters, 1313 (1969); A.K.
      Banerjee and M. Gut, J. Org. Chem., 34,
      1614 (1969); J. Knabe, H. Junginger, W.
      Geismar, and H. Wolf, Ann. Chem., 739, 15
      (1970); D.G. Neilson, U. Zakir, and C.M.
      Scrimgeour, J. Chem. Soc. (C), 898 (1971).
123. G. Snatzke, H. Ripperger, C. Horstmann, and
      K. Schreiber, Tetrahedron, 22, 3103 (1966);
      H. Wolf, Tetrahedron Letters, 1075 (1965);
      5151 (1966); M. Legrand and R. Bucourt,
      Bull. Soc. Chim. France, 2241 (1967); F.I.
      Carroll, A. Sobti, and R. Meck, Tetra-
      hedron Letters, 405 (1971).
124. M. Gorodetsky, N. Danieli, and Y. Mazur,
      J. Org. Chem., 32, 760 (1967); O. Červinka
      and L. Hub, Collect. Czech. Chem. Comm.,
      33, 2927 (1968); T. Sasaki and S. Eguchi,
      Bull. Chem. Soc. Japan, 41, 2453 (1968);
      D. Lavie, I. Kirson, E. Glotter, and G.
      Snatzke, Tetrahedron, 26, 2221 (1970); O.
      Korver, Tetrahedron, 26, 2391 (1970); W.
      Stöcklin, T.G. Waddell, and T.A. Geissman,
      Tetrahedron, 26, 2397 (1970); M.J. Brienne
      and J. Jacques, Tetrahedron, 26, 5087
      (1970); T. Suga, T. Hirata, M. Noda, and T.
      Matsuura, Experientia, 26, 1192 (1970).
125. A.F. Beecham, Tetrahedron Letters, 2355,
      3591 (1968); 4897 (1969); A.F. Beecham and
      R.R. Sauers, Tetrahedron Letters, 4763 (1970).

126. J.P. Jennings, W. Klyne, W.P. Mose, and P.
     M. Scopes, Chem. Comm., 553 (1966); J.P.
     Jennings, W.P. Mose, and P.M. Scopes, J.
     Chem. Soc. (C), 1102 (1967).
127. W. Gaffield and W.G. Galetto, Tetrahedron,
     27, 915 (1971).
128. P.M. Scopes, R.N. Thomas, and M.B. Rahman,
     J. Chem. Soc., 1671 (1971).
129. U. Weiss and H. Ziffer, J. Org. Chem., 28,
     1248 (1963); P.F. Wareing and G. Ryback,
     Endeavour, 29, 84 (1970); J. Cymerman Craig,
     W.E. Pereira, B. Halpern, and J.W. Westley,
     Tetrahedron, 27, 1173 (1971).
130. G. Snatzke, M. Schwang, and P. Welzel, in
     Some Newer Physical Methods in Structural
     Chemistry, Mass Spectrometry, Optical Ro-
     tatory Dispersion, and Circular Dichroism,
     B. Bonnett and J.G. Davis (edit.), United
     Trade Press Ltd., London (1967); T.G. Wad-
     dell, W. Stöcklin, and T.A. Geissman, Tetra-
     hedron Letters, 1313 (1969); W. Rosenbrook
     and R.E. Carney, Tetrahedron Letters, 1867
     (1970); W. Herz, K. Aota, and A.L. Hall, J.
     Org. Chem., 35, 4117 (1970); G.A. Ellestad,
     R.H. Evans, M.P. Kunstmann, J.E. Lancaster,
     and G.O. Morton, J. Amer. Chem. Soc., 92,
     5483 (1970).
131. G. Montaudo and C.G. Overberger, J. Amer.
     Chem. Soc., 91, 753 (1969).
132. M. Kasha, J. Radiation Res., 20, 55 (1963).
133. C. Toniolo, V. Perciaccante, J. Falcetta,
     R. Rupp, and M. Goodman, J. Org. Chem., 35,
     6 (1970).
134. G. Snatzke and E. Otto, Tetrahedron, 25,
     2041 (1969).
135. C. Djerassi, E. Lund, E. Bunnenberg, and J.
     C. Sheehan, J. Org. Chem., 26, 4509 (1961);
     F.A. Mikulski, Ph.D. Thesis, Princeton Uni-
     versity (1965); D.T. Witiak, Z. Muhi-Eldeen,
     N. Mahishi, O.P. Sethi, and M.C. Gerald, J.
     Med. Chem., 14, 24 (1971).

136. W. Gaffield, Chem. and Ind., 1460 (1964);
     J. Cymerman Craig and S.K. Roy, Tetrahedron,
     21, 391 (1965); M. Legrand and R. Viennet,
     Bull. Soc. Chim. France, 679 (1965); 2798
     (1966); R.D. Anand and M.K. Hargreaves,
     Chem. and Ind., 880 (1968); J. Horwitz, E.
     H. Strickland, and C. Billups, J. Amer.
     Chem. Soc., 91, 184 (1969); D.G. Neilson,
     I.A. Khan, and R.S. Whitehead, J. Chem.
     Soc. (C), 1853 (1968); J.M. Tsangaris, J.
     Wen Chang, and R.B. Martin, J. Amer. Chem.
     Soc., 91, 726 (1969); L. Fowden, P.M.
     Scopes, and R.N. Thomas, J. Chem. Soc. (C),
     833 (1971).
137. L.I. Katzin and E. Gulyas, J. Amer. Chem.
     Soc., 90, 247 (1968).
138. E.C. Jorgensen, Tetrahedron Letters, 863
     (1971).
139. Y.P. Myer and L.H. MacDonald, J. Amer.
     Chem. Soc., 89, 7142 (1967); I. Frič, V.
     Spiro, and K. Blaha, Coll. Czech. Chem.
     Comm., 33, 4008 (1968); H. Wyler and J.
     Chiovini, Helv. Chim. Acta, 51, 1476 (1968);
     N. Sakota, K. Okita, and Y. Matsui, Bull.
     Chem. Soc. Japan, 43, 1138 (1970); O.
     Cervinka, L. Hub, and G. Snatzke, Coll.
     Czechosl. Chem. Comm., 36, 1687 (1971).
140. G. Barth, W. Voelter, E. Bunnenberg, and
     C. Djerassi, Chem. Comm., 355 (1969); O.
     Korver, Tetrahedron, 26, 5507 (1970).
141. D.L. Dull and H.S. Mosher, J. Amer. Chem.
     Soc., 89, 4230 (1967); J. Cymerman Craig
     and W.E. Pereira, Tetrahedron Letters, 1563
     (1970); Tetrahedron, 26, 3457 (1970); G.
     Barth, W. Voelter, H.S. Mosher, E. Bunnen-
     berg, and C. Djerassi, J. Amer. Chem. Soc.,
     92, 875 (1970); I. Listowsky, G. Avigad,
     and S. Englard, J. Org. Chem., 35, 1080
     (1970).
142. W. Thiemann, Tetrahedron, 27, 1465 (1971).
143. W. Voelter, E. Bayer, G. Barth, E. Bunnen-
     berg, and C. Djerassi, Chem. Ber., 102, 2003
     (1969).

144. L.I. Katzin and E. Gulyas, J. Amer. Chem. Soc., 91, 6940 (1969).

145. J.M. Tsangaris and R.B. Martin, J. Amer. Chem. Soc., 92, 4255 (1970); C.J. Hawkins and C.L. Wong, Austral. J. Chem., 23, 2237 (1970).

146. M.H. Ghandehari, T.N. Andersen, D.R. Boone, and H. Eyring, J. Amer. Chem. Soc., 92, 6466 (1970); K. Kawasaki, J. Yoshi, and M. Shibata, Bull. Chem. Soc. Japan, 43, 3819 (1970).

147. P. Crabbé and L. Pinelo, Chem. and Ind., 158 (1966); G.G. Lyle and R. Mestrallet Barrera, J. Org. Chem., 29, 3311 (1964); P. Crabbé, Ind. Chim. Belg., 33, 87 (1968).

148. P. Crabbé and W. Klyne, Tetrahedron, 23, 3449 (1967).

149. G.G. DeAngelis and W.C. Wildman, Tetrahedron, 25, 5099 (1969).

150. J.H. Brewster and J.G. Buta, J. Amer. Chem. Soc., 88, 2233 (1966); L. Verbit, A.S. Rao, and J.W. Clark-Lewis, Tetrahedron, 24, 5839 (1968).

151. K. Kuriyama, T. Iwata, M. Moriyama, K. Kotera, Y. Hamada, R. Mitsui, and K. Takeda, J. Chem. Soc. (B), 46 (1967).

152. K. Mislow, M.A.W. Glass, R.E. O'Brien, P. Rutkin, D.H. Steinberg, J. Weiss, and C. Djerassi, J. Amer. Chem. Soc., 84, 1455 (1962); K. Mislow, E. Bunnenberg, R. Records, K. Wellman, and C. Djerassi, J. Amer. Chem. Soc., 85, 1342 (1963); K. Mislow, M.A.W. Glass, H.B. Hopps, E. Simon, and G.H. Wahl, J. Amer. Chem. Soc., 86, 1710 (1964); T.R. Hollands, P. de Mayo, M. Nisbet, and P. Crabbé, Canad. J. Chem., 43, 3008 (1965); J.M. Insole, J. Chem. Soc., (C), 1712 (1971), and references cited therein.

153. G.G. Lyle and M.J. Piazza, J. Org. Chem., 33, 2478 (1968).

154. D.W. Miles, R.K. Robins, and H. Eyring, J. Phys. Chem., 71, 3931 (1967).

155.   H. Wynberg, Acc. Chem. Res., 4, 65 (1971);
       R.H. Martin, M. Flammang-Barbieux, J.P.
       Cosyn, and M. Gelbcke, Tetrahedron Letters,
       3507 (1968); H. Wynberg and M.B. Groen, J.
       Amer. Chem. Soc., 90, 5339 (1968); Chem.
       Comm., 964 (1969); J. Amer. Chem. Soc., 92,
       6664 (1970); 93, 2968 (1971); R.H. Martin,
       M.J. Marchant, and M. Baes, Helv. Chim.
       Acta, 54, 358 (1971).
156.   G. Snatzke and P.C. Ho, Tetrahedron, 27,
       3645 (1971).
157.   R.S. Cahn, C. Ingold, and V. Prelog, Angew.
       Chem. Int. Edit., 5, 385 (1966); M.B.
       Groen, G. Stulen, G.J. Visser, and H.
       Wynberg, J. Amer. Chem. Soc., 92, 7218
       (1970), specially footnote 9.
158.   S.F. Mason and G.W. Vane, J. Chem. Soc.
       (B), 370 (1966); S.F. Mason, G.W. Vane, K.
       Schofield, R.J. Wells, and J.S. Whitehurst,
       J. Chem. Soc. (B), 553 (1967).
159.   G. Snatzke and G. Eckhardt, in Experimen-
       tal Methods in Molecular Biology, Cl.
       Nicolau (edit.), in press.
160.   L. Verbit, J. Amer. Chem. Soc., 87, 1617
       (1965); 88, 5340 (1966); P. Crabbé, P.
       Demoen, and P. Janssen, Bull. Soc. Chim.
       France, 2855 (1965); L. Verbit, S. Mitsui,
       and Y. Senda, Tetrahedron, 22, 753 (1966);
       L. Verbit and P.J. Heffron, Tetrahedron,
       23, 3865 (1967); L. Verbit, E. Pfeil, and
       W. Becker, Tetrahedron Letters, 2169 (1967);
       L. Verbit and P.J. Heffron, Tetrahedron,
       24, 1231 (1968); L. Verbit, A.S. Rao, and
       J.W. Clark-Lewis, Tetrahedron, 24, 5839
       (1968); I. Moretti and G. Torre, Tetra-
       hedron Letters, 2717 (1969).
161.   H. Brockmann and M. Legrand, Tetrahedron,
       19, 395 (1963); H. Brockmann, H. Brockmann,
       and J. Niemeyer, Tetrahedron Letters, 4719
       (1968); L.A. Mitscher, A.C. Bonacci, and
       T.D. Sokoloski, Tetrahedron Letters, 5361
       (1968); L.A. Mitscher, J.V. Juvarkar, Wm.
       Rosenbrook, W.W. Andres, J. Schenck, and
       R.S. Egan, J. Amer. Chem. Soc., 92, 6070
       (1970).

162. W. Gaffield and A.C. Waiss, Chem. Comm.,29
      (1968); K.R. Markham and T.J. Mabry, Tetra-
      hedron, 24, 823 (1968); L. Verbit and J.W.
      Clark-Lewis, Tetrahedron, 24, 5519 (1968);
      K. Kurosawa, W.D. Ollis, B.T. Redman, I.O.
      Sutherland, O.R. Gottlieb, and H. Magalhães,
      Chem. Comm., 1265 (1968); W.D. Ollis, C.A.
      Rhodes, and I.O. Sutherland, Tetrahedron,
      23, 4741 (1967); H. Arakawa, N. Torimoto,
      and Y. Masui, Tetrahedron Letters, 4115
      (1968); W. Gaffield, Tetrahedron, 26, 4093
      (1970); G. Aurnhammer, H. Wagner, L. Hör-
      hammer, and L. Farkas, Chem. Ber., 103,
      3667 (1970); K.K. Purushothaman, V.M.
      Kishore, V. Narayanaswami, and J.D. Con-
      nolly, J. Chem. Soc., (C), 2420 (1971).
163. D.C. Ayres, J.A. Harris, and P.B. Hulbert,
      J. Chem. Soc., (C), 1111 (1971), and refer-
      ences therein.
164. U. Kuffner and K. Schlögl, Tetrahedron Let-
      ters, 1773 (1971).
165. J. Trojánek, Z. Koblikova, and K. Bláha,
      Coll. Czech. Chem. Comm., 33, 2950 (1968).
166. W. Klyne, R.J. Swan, A.A. Gorman, A.
      Guggisberg, and H. Schmid, Helv. Chim. Acta,
      51, 1168 (1968).
167. T. Kametani and M. Ihara, J. Chem. Soc.
      (C), 1305 (1968); G. Snatzke, J. Hrbek, L.
      Hruban, A. Horeau, and F. Šantavý, Tetra-
      hedron, 26, 5013 (1970).
168. K. Kotera, Y. Hamada, and R. Mitsui, Tetra-
      hedron, 24, 2463 (1968).
169. T. Kametani, H. Sugi, and S. Shibuya, Tetra-
      hedron, 27, 2409 (1971) and references
      cited.
170. J.P. Ferris, C.B. Boyce, and R.C. Briner,
      J. Amer. Chem. Soc., 93, 2942 (1971); J.P.
      Ferris, C.B. Boyce, R.C. Briner, U. Weiss,
      I.H. Qureshi, and N.E. Sharpless, J. Amer.
      Chem. Soc., 93, 2963 (1971).
171. R.T. Lalonde, E. Auer, C. Fook Wong, and
      V.P. Muralidharan, J. Amer. Chem. Soc., 93,
      2501 (1971).

172. F. Šantavy, P. Sedmera, G. Snatzke, and T. Reinstein, Helv. Chim. Acta, 54, 1084 (1971).

173. H. Carpio, A. Cervantes, and P. Crabbé, Bull. Soc. Chim. France, 1256 (1969).

174. W.S. Chilton and R.C. Krahn, J. Amer. Chem. Soc., 90, 1318 (1968); K. Yoshihira, M. Tezuka, and S. Natori, Tetrahedron Letters, 7 (1970); J. Karliner and E. Yee, J. Heter. Chem., 7, 1109 (1970); G. Gottarelli and B. Samori, Tetrahedron Letters, 2055 (1970); E. Dornhege and G. Snatzke, Tetrahedron, 26, 3059 (1970); H.E. Smith and A.A. Hicks, Chem. Comm., 1112 (1970); G. Haas, P.B. Hulbert, W. Klyne, V. Prelog, and G. Snatzke, Helv. Chim. Acta, 54, 491 (1971).

175. S. Hagishita and K. Kuriyama, Bull. Chem. Soc. Japan, 44, 617 (1971); 44, 2177 (1971).

176. N. Harada and K. Nakanishi, J. Amer. Chem. Soc., 90, 7351 (1968).

177. S. Marumo, H. Harada, K. Nakanishi, and T. Nishida, Chem. Comm., 1693 (1970).

178. N. Harada and K. Nakanishi, J. Amer. Chem. Soc., 91, 3989 (1969); M. Koreeda, N. Harada, and K. Nakanishi, Chem. Comm., 548 (1969); N. Harada, K. Nakanishi, and S. Tatsuoka, J. Amer. Chem. Soc., 91, 5896 (1969); N. Harada and K. Nakanishi, Chem. Comm., 310 (1970).

179. G. Snatzke, G. Wollenberg, J. Hrbek, F. Šantavý, K. Bláha, W. Klyne, and R.J. Swan, Tetrahedron, 25, 5059 (1969).

180. P. Crabbé, Chem. and Ind., 917 (1969).

181. W.L. Bencze, B. Kisis, R.T. Puckett, and N. Finch, Tetrahedron, 26, 5407 (1970).

182. D.E. Bays, R.C. Cookson, R.R. Hill, J.F. McGhie, and G.E. Usher, J. Chem. Soc., 1563 (1964).

183. A.H. Haines and C.S.P. Jenkins, J. Chem. Soc., (C), 1438 (1971).

184. J. Parello and F. Picot, Tetrahedron Letters, 5083 (1968).

185. C. Toniolo, Tetrahedron, 26, 5479 (1970).

186. C. Djerassi, E. Lund, E. Bunnenberg, and
     B. Sjöberg, J. Amer. Chem. Soc., 83, 2307
     (1961); G. Snatzke, H. Ripperger, C. Horst-
     mann, and K. Schreiber, Tetrahedron, 22,
     3103 (1966); A. La Manna and V. Ghislandi,
     II Farmaco, 17, 355 (1962).
187. S. Mitchell, J. Chem. Soc., 3258 (1928);
     1829 (1930); S. Mitchell and S.B. Cormack,
     J. Chem. Soc., 415 (1932).
188. W. Kuhn and H.L. Lehmann, Z. physik. Chem.,
     B18, 32 (1932); W. Kuhn and H. Biller, Z.
     physik, Chem., B19, 1 (1935); H.B. Elkins
     and W. Kuhn, J. Amer. Chem. Soc., 57, 296
     (1935); W. Kuhn, Ann. Rev. Phys. Chem., 9,
     417 (1958).
189. F. Nerdel, K. Becker, and C. Kresze, Chem.
     Ber., 89, 2862 (1956); G. Dudek, J. Org.
     Chem., 32, 2016 (1967).
190. A.P. Terentev and V.M. Potapov, Zh. Obschch.
     Khim., 28, 1161, 3323 (1958); V.M. Potapov,
     A.P. Terentev, and R.I. Sarylaeva, Zh.
     Obschch. Khim., 29, 3139 (1959); V.M.
     Potapov and A.P. Terentev, Zh. Obschch.
     Khim., 30, 666 (1960); V.M. Potapov, A.P.
     Terentev, and S.P. Spivak, Zh. Obschch.
     Khim., 31, 2415 (1961).
191. H.E. Smith, S.L. Cook, and M.E. Warren,
     J. Org. Chem., 29, 2265 (1964).
192. H.E. Smith, M.E. Warren, and A.W. Ingersoll,
     J. Amer. Chem. Soc., 84, 1513 (1962).
193. D. Bertin and M. Legrand, Compt. rend.,
     256, 960 (1963); M.E. Warren and H.E. Smith,
     J. Amer. Chem. Soc., 87, 1757 (1965); H.E.
     Smith and T.Ch. Willis, J. Org. Chem., 30,
     2654 (1965); H. Ripperger, K. Schreiber,
     G. Snatzke, and K. Heller, Z. Chem., 5, 62
     (1965); H.E. Smith and R. Records, Tetra-
     hedron, 22, 813 (1966); H. Ripperger, K.
     Schreiber, G. Snatzke, and K. Ponsold,
     Tetrahedron, 25, 827 (1969); H.E. Smith and
     T.C. Willis, Tetrahedron, 26, 107 (1970).

194. J.H. Brewster and S.F. Osman, J. Amer.
     Chem. Soc., 82, 5754 (1960); C. Djerassi,
     E. Lund, E. Bunnenberg, and J.C. Sheehan,
     J. Org. Chem., 26, 4509 (1961); H. Wolf,
     E. Bunnenberg, and C. Djerassi, Chem. Ber.,
     97, 533 (1964).
195. A. La Manna and V. Ghislandi, Il Farmaco,
     19, 480 (1964).
196. A. La Manna, V. Ghislandi, P.M. Scopes,
     and R.H. Swan, Il Farmaco, 20, 842 (1965).
197. B. Sjöberg, B. Karlen, and R. Dahlbom,
     Acta Chem. Scand., 16, 1071 (1962); S. Ya-
     mada, K. Ishikawa, and K. Achiwa, Chem.
     Pharm. Bull. Japan, 13, 1266 (1965); E.
     Bach, A. Kjaer, R. Dahlbom, T. Walle, B.
     Sjöberg, E. Bunnenberg, C. Djerassi, and
     R. Records, Acta. Chem. Scand., 20, 2781
     (1966).
198. G.C. Barrett and A.R. Khokhar, J. Chem.
     Soc. (C), 1120 (1969); G.C. Barrett, J.
     Chem. Soc. (C), 1123 (1969).
199. C. Djerassi, H. Wolf, and E. Bunnenberg,
     J. Amer. Chem. Soc., 84, 4552 (1962); C.
     Djerassi, K. Undheim, R.C. Sheppard, W.G.
     Terry, and B. Sjöberg, Acta. Chem. Scand.,
     15, 903 (1961).
200. V.N. Potapov, V.N. Demyanovich, and A.P.
     Terentev, Vestn. Mosk. Univ. Ser. II,
     Khim., 20, 56 (1965); Chem. Abst., 62,
     14461 (1965).
201. P. Crabbé, B. Halpern, and E. Santos, Tetra-
     hedron, 24, 4299 (1968); G. Aguilar-Santos,
     E. Santos, and P. Crabbé, J. Org. Chem.,
     32, 2642 (1967); E. Santos, J. Padilla,
     and P. Crabbé, Canad. J. Chem., 45, 2275
     (1967); V. Tortorella, G. Bettoni, B. Hal-
     pern, and P. Crabbé, in preparation.
202. P. Crabbé, B. Halpern, and E. Santos,
     Tetrahedron, 24, 4315 (1968).
203. A.H. Beckett and L.G. Brookes, Tetrahedron,
     24, 1283 (1968); H.E. Smith, M.E. Warren,
     and L.I. Katzin, Tetrahedron, 24, 1327
     (1968); A. La Manna, V. Ghislandi, P.B.
     Hulbert, and P.M. Scopes, Il Farmaco, 23,
     1161 (1968).

204. H.E. Smith and T.C. Willis, J. Amer. Chem. Soc., 93, 2282 (1971).

205. J.H. Brewster and J.G. Buta, J. Amer. Chem. Soc., 88, 2233 (1966).

206. U. Nagai and M. Kurumi, Chem. Pharm. Bull. Japan, 18, 831 (1970).

207. W.S. Briggs and C. Djerassi, Tetrahedron, 21, 3455 (1965); I.P. Dirkx and T.J. de Boer, Rec. Trav. Chim., 83, 535 (1964).

208. H. Ripperger, K. Schreiber, and F.J. Sych, J. prakt. Chem., 312, 471 (1970); H. Ripperger, Tetrahedron, 25, 725 (1969); H. Ripperger, Angew. Chem. Int. Edit., 6, 704 (1967).

209. C. Djerassi, A. Moscowitz, K. Ponsold, and G. Steiner, J. Amer. Chem. Soc., 89, 347 (1967); W.D. Closson and H.B. Gray, J. Amer. Chem. Soc., 85, 290 (1963); E. Lieber, J.S. Curtice, and C.N.R. Rao, Chem. and Ind., 586 (1966); K. Kischa and E. Zbiral, Tetrahedron, 26, 1417 (1970).

210. H. Paulsen, Chem. Ber., 101, 1571 (1968).

211. H. Ripperger, K. Schreiber, and G. Snatzke, Tetrahedron, 21, 1027 (1965), and references cited; Z. Badr, R. Bonnett, T.R. Emerson, and W. Klyne, J. Chem. Soc., 4503 (1965); R. Bonnett and T.R. Emerson, J. Chem. Soc., 4508 (1965); Z. Badr, R. Bonnett, W. Klyne, R.J. Swan, and J. Wood, J. Chem. Soc. (C), 2047 (1966).

212. H. Ripperger and K. Schreiber, Tetrahedron, 23, 1841 (1967); H. Ripperger and H. Pracejus, Tetrahedron, 24, 99 (1968).

213. H. Ripperger, K. Schreiber, and G. Snatzke, Tetrahedron, 21, 727 (1965), and references therein.

214. H. Ripperger and K. Schreiber, J. Prakt. Chem., in press.

215. G. Snatzke, D. Becher, and J.R. Bull, Tetrahedron, 20, 2443 (1964); G. Snatzke, J. Chem. Soc., 5002 (1965); J.R. Bull, J.P. Jennings, W. Klyne, G.D. Meakins, P.M. Scopes, and G. Snatzke, J. Chem. Soc., 3152 (1965).

216. G. Snatzke and J. Himmelreich, Tetrahedron, 23, 4337 (1967); J. Buckingham and R.D. Guthrie, J. Chem. Soc., (C), 1939 (1969); 106 (1970); D.J. Severn and E.M. Kosower, J. Amer. Chem. Soc., 91, 1710 (1969); G. Snatzke, Riechst. Arom. Körperfl., 19, 98 (1969); M. Suchy, L. Dolejs, V. Herout, V. Sorm, G. Snatzke, and J. Himmelreich, Coll. Czech. Chem. Comm., 34, 229 (1969); W. Herz, K. Aota, M. Holub, and Z. Zamek, J. Org. Chem., 35, 2611 (1970); G. Snatzke, H. Langen, and J. Himmerlreich, Ann. Chem., 744, 142 (1971).

217. G. Snatzke, H. Laurent, and R. Wiechert, Tetrahedron, 25, 761 (1969).

218. R.G. Kostyanovsky, Z.E. Samojlova, and I.I. Tchervin, Tetrahedron Letters, 719 (1969).

219. C. Djerassi, D.A. Lightner, D.A. Schooley, K. Takeda, T. Komeno, and K. Kuriyama, Tetrahedron, 24, 6913 (1968).

220. T.M. Lowry and H. Hudson, Phil. Trans. Roy. Soc. (London), 232A, 117 (1933); C. Djerassi, H. Wolf, and E. Bunnenberg, J. Amer. Chem. Soc., 84, 4552 (1962); B. Sjöberg, D.J. Cram, L. Wolf, and C. Djerassi, Acta Chem. Scand., 16, 1079 (1962); Y. Tsuzuki, K. Tanabe, M. Akagi, and S. Tejima, Bull. Chem. Soc. Japan, 40, 628 (1967).

221. B. Sjöberg, A. Fredga, and C. Djerassi, J. Amer. Chem. Soc., 81, 5002 (1959).

222. D. Adinarayana, et al. J. Chem. Soc. (C), 29 (1971), and references therein.

223. C. Djerassi and K. Undheim, J. Amer. Chem. Soc., 82, 5755 (1960); C. Djerassi, K. Undheim, and A.M. Weidler, Acta Chem. Scand., 16, 1147 (1962).

224. P. Laur, H. Häuser, J.E. Gurst, and K. Mislow, J. Org. Chem., 32, 498 (1967); P. Salvadori, Chem. Comm., 1203 (1968).

225. A. Fredga, Acta Chem. Scand., 4, 1307 (1950); C. Djerassi, A. Fredga, and B. Sjöberg, Acta Chem. Scand., 15, 417 (1961); C. Djerassi, H. Wolf, and E. Bunnenberg, J. Amer. Chem. Soc., 84, 4552 (1962); A.F.

Beecham and A. McL. Mathieson, Tetrahedron Letters, 3139 (1966).

226. R.C. Cookson, G.H. Cooper, and J. Hudec, J. Chem. Soc. (B), 1004 (1967).

227. C. Djerassi and D. Herbst, J. Org. Chem., 26, 4675 (1961); R.E. Ballard and S.F. Mason, J. Chem. Soc., 1624 (1963); P. Pino, C. Carlini, E. Chiellini, F. Ciardelli, and P. Salvadori, J. Amer. Chem. Soc., 90, 5025 (1968).

228. N.M. Green, W.P. Mose, and P.M. Scopes, J. Chem. Soc. (C), 1330 (1970); P. Salvadori, Chem. Comm., 1203 (1968); P. Laur, H. Häuser, J.E. Gurst, and K. Mislow, J. Org. Chem., 32, 498 (1967).

229. K.K. Andersen, W. Gaffield, N.E. Papanikolaou, J.W. Foley, and R.I. Perkins, J. Amer. Chem. Soc., 86, 5637 (1964); K. Mislow, Angew. Chem. Intern. Edit., 4, 717 (1965); K. Mislow, M.M. Green, and M. Raban, J. Amer. Chem. Soc., 87, 2761 (1965); C.R. Johnson and D. McCants, J. Amer. Chem. Soc., 87, 5404 (1965); K. Mislow, Rec. Chem. Progress, 28, 217 (1967); S.I. Goldberg and M.S. Sahli, J. Org. Chem., 32, 2059 (1967); R. Nagarajan, B.H. Chollar, and R.M. Dodson, Chem. Comm., 550 (1967); P.B. Sollman, R. Nagarajan, and R.M. Dodson, Chem. Comm., 552 (1967); D.N. Jones, M.J. Green, M.A. Saeed, and R.D. Whitehouse, Chem. Comm., 1003 (1967); D.N. Jones and M.J. Green, J. Chem. Soc. (C), 532 (1967); M. Axelrod, P. Bickart, M.L. Goldstein, M.M. Green, A. Kjaer, and K. Mislow, Tetrahedron Letters, 3249 (1968); D.N. Jones, M.J. Green, and R.D. Whitehouse, Chem. Comm., 1634 (1968); D.N. Jones, M.J. Green, M.A. Saeed, and R.D. Whitehouse, J. Chem. Soc. (C), 1362 (1968); D.N. Jones, M.J. Green, and R.D. Whitehouse, J. Chem. Soc. (C), 1166 (1969); D.N. Jones and W. Higgins, J. Chem. Soc. (C), 2159 (1969); M. Mikolajczyk and M. Para, Chem. Comm., 1192 (1969); P.D. Henson and K. Mislow, Chem. Comm., 413 (1969); D.N.

Jones and W. Higgins, J. Chem. Soc. (C), 81 (1970); M. Cinquini, St. Colonna, I. Moretti, and G. Torre, Tetrahedron Letters, 2773 (1970).

230. M.K. Hargreaves, P.G. Modi, and J.G. Pritchard, Chem. Comm., 1306 (1968), and references therein.

231. D.N. Jones, D. Mundy, and R.D. Whitehouse, Chem. Comm., 1636 (1968); D.N. Jones, D. Mundy, and R.D. Whitehouse, J. Chem. Soc. (C), 1668 (1969); D.N. Jones, E. Helmy, and A.C.F. Edmonds, J. Chem. Soc. (C), 833 (1970).

232. C.H. Robinson, L. Milewich, G. Snatzke, W. Klyne, and S.R. Wallis, J. Chem. Soc. (C), 1245 (1968).

233. D.J. Cram, J. Day, D.R. Rayner, D.M. von Schriltz, D.J. Duchamp, and D.C. Garwood, J. Amer. Chem. Soc., 92, 7369 (1970).

234. M. Raban and S.K. Lauderback, J. Amer. Chem. Soc., 93, 2781 (1971).

235. O. Korpium and K. Mislow, J. Amer. Chem. Soc., 89, 4784 (1967); R.A. Lewis, O. Korpium, and K. Mislow, J. Amer. Chem. Soc., 89, 4786 (1967); W.D. Balzer, Tetrahedron Letters, 1189 (1968); F.D. Saeva, D.R. Rayner, and K. Mislow, J. Amer. Chem. Soc., 90, 4176 (1968).

236. J. Riess, Bull. Soc. Chim. France, 18, 29, 3552 (1965); J. Riess and C. Ourisson, Bull. Soc. Chim. France, 933 (1965); L. Horner, J.P. Bercz, and C.V. Bercz, Tetrahedron Letters, 5783 (1966); D. Hellwinkel, Chem. Ber., 99, 3642 (1966); R.A. Lewis, O. Korpium, and K. Mislow, J. Amer. Chem. Soc., 89, 4786 (1967); W.D. Balzer, Tetrahedron Letters, 1189 (1968); C. Donninger and D.H. Hutson, Tetrahedron Letters, 4871 (1968); F.H. Westheimer, Acc. Chem. Res., 1, 70 (1968); J.N. Seiber and H. Tolkmith, Tetrahedron, 25, 381 (1969); K. Mislow, Acc. Chem. Res., 3, 321 (1970); W.B. Farnham, R.K. Murray, and K. Mislow, J. Amer. Chem. Soc., 92, 5809 (1970); D. Hellwinkel

and S.F. Mason, J. Chem. Soc. (B), 640
(1970); O. Červinka, O. Bělovský, and M.
Hepnerová, Chem. Comm., 562 (1970); I.J.
Borowitz, K.C. Kirby, P.E. Rusek, and E.W.
R. Casper, J. Org. Chem., 36, 88 (1971).

237. C.G. Overberger and J.K. Weise, J. Amer.
Chem. Soc., 90, 3525, 3538 (1968).

238. R. Rahman, S. Safe, and A. Taylor, Quart.
Reviews, 24, 208 (1970); H. Herrmann, R.
Hodges, and A. Taylor, J. Chem. Soc., 4315
(1964); A.F. Beecham, J. Fridrichsons, and
A. McL. Mathieson, Tetrahedron Letters,
3131 (1966); A.F. Beecham and A. McL.
Mathieson, Tetrahedron Letters, 3139
(1966); M. Carmack and L.A. Neubert, J.
Amer. Chem. Soc., 89, 7134 (1967); A.F.
Beecham, J.W. Loder, and G.B. Russell,
Tetrahedron Letters, 1785 (1968); J.A.
Barltrop, P.M. Hayes, and M. Calvin, J.
Amer. Chem. Soc., 76, 4348 (1954); R.M.
Dodson and V.C. Nelson, J. Org. Chem., 33,
3966 (1968); G. Claeson, Acta Chem. Scand.,
22, 2429 (1968); P.C. Kahn and S. Beychok,
J. Amer. Chem. Soc., 90, 4168 (1968); R.
Nagarajan, N. Neuss, and M.M. Marsh, J.
Amer. Chem. Soc., 90, 6518 (1968); S. Safe
and A. Taylor, Chem. Comm., 1466 (1969);
K.C. Murdock and R.B. Angier, Chem. Comm.,
55 (1970); D. Hauser, H.P. Weber, and H.P.
Sigg, Helv. Chim. Acta, 53, 1061 (1970).

239. C.G. Overberger, G. Montaudo, J. Šebenda,
and R.A. Veneski, J. Amer. Chem. Soc., 91,
1256 (1969); H. Edelhoch, R.E. Lippoldt,
and M. Wilchek, J. Biol. Chem., 243, 4799
(1968).

240. P. Salvadori, L. Lardicci, and P. Pino,
Tetrahedron Letters, 1641 (1965); P. Salva-
dori, L. Lardicci, G. Consiglio, and P.
Pino, Tetrahedron Letters, 5343 (1966); P.
Vink, C. Blomberg, A.D. Vreugdenhil, and
F. Bickelhaupt, Tetrahedron Letters, 6419
(1966); J.S. Baran, J. Med. Chem., 10, 1039
(1967); W. Klyne, W.P. Mose, P.M. Scopes,
G.M. Holder, and W.B. Whalley, J. Chem.
Soc. (C), 1273 (1967); S.F. Mason and G.W.

Vane, Chem. Comm., 598 (1967).

241. R.W. Murray, R.D. Youssefyeh, and P.R. Story, J. Amer. Chem. Soc., 88, 3655 (1966).

242. Y. Brunel, H. Lemaire, and A. Rassat, Bull. Soc. Chim. France, 1895 (1964).

243. J. Parello and X. Lusinchi, Tetrahedron, 24, 6747 (1968).

244. J. Parello, R. Beugelmans, P. Millet, and X. Lusinchi, Tetrahedron Letters, 5087 (1968).

245. N.D. Vietmeyer and C. Djerassi, J. Org. Chem., 35, 3591 (1970).

246. W.J. McGahren and M.P. Kunstmann, J. Amer. Chem. Soc., 92, 1587 (1970).

247. R.C. Pandey, V.F. German, Y. Nishikawa, et al. J. Amer. Chem. Soc., 93, 3738 (1971).

248. W. Meister, R.D. Guthrie, J.L. Maxwell, D.A. Jaeger, and D.J. Cram, J. Amer. Chem. Soc., 91, 4452 (1969).

249. N.J. Greenfield and G.D. Fasman, J. Amer. Chem. Soc., 92, 177 (1970).

250. K. Isono, K. Asahi, and S. Suzuki, J. Amer. Chem. Soc., 91, 7490 (1969).

251. R. Nagarajan and D.O. Spry, J. Amer. Chem. Soc., 93, 2310 (1971).

252. L. Bartlett, W. Klyne, W.P. Mose, P.M. Scopes, G. Galasko, A.K. Mallams, B.C.L. Weedon, J. Szabolcs, and G. Tóth, J. Chem. Soc. (C), 2527 (1969); C.H. Eugster, R. Buchecker, Ch. Tscharner, G. Uhde, and G. Ohloff, Helv. Chim. Acta, 52, 1729 (1969); R. Buchecker, H. Yokoyama, and C.H. Eugster, Helv. Chim. Acta, 53, 1210 (1970); C.H. Eugster, Angew. Chem., 82, 259 (1970); D. Goodfellow, G.P. Moss, and B.C.L. Weedon, Chem. Comm., 1578 (1970); R. Buchecker and C.H. Eugster, Helv. Chim. Acta, 54, 327 (1971).

253. R. Corriu, J. Masse, and G. Royo, Compt. rend., 264, 987 (1964); L.H. Sommer and R. Mason, J. Amer. Chem. Soc., 87, 1619 (1965); L. Spialter and D.H. O'Brien, J. Org. Chem., 31, 3048 (1966); K. Bláha, I. Frič, and H.D. Jakubke, Coll. Czech. Chem. Comm., 32,

558 (1967); L.H. Sommer and J. McLick, J. Amer. Chem. Soc., 89, 5806 (1967); 91, 2001 (1969); C. Eaborn, R.E.E. Hill, and P. Simpson, Chem. Comm., 1077 (1968); R. Corriu and G. Lanneau, Compt. rend., 267, 782 (1968); P.A. Hart and M.P. Tripp, Chem. Comm., 174 (1969); D.N. Jones, D. Mundy, and R.D. Whitehouse, Chem. Comm., 86 (1970); A. Jean and M. Lequan, Tetrahedron Letters, 1517 (1970); R. Corriu and J. Masse, Tetrahedron, 26, 5123 (1970); H. Kessler, Naturwiss., 58, 46 (1971).

III. SOLVENT AND TEMPERATURE EFFECTS

Solute-solvent interactions manifest them-
selves in many spectroscopic measurements, including the chiroptical methods. In fact, modification of the nature of the solvent can affect
the Cotton effect, since new factors are intro-
duced, such as solute-solvent complex formation,
dipole-dipole interaction, hydrogen bonding, conformational equilibria, charge-transfer, etc.
(12-15,254). To some extent this is observed in
the case of D-(+)-camphor ($\underline{1}$), which shows a +64
in ethanol, a +69 in dioxane, and a +73 in hex-
ane solution. Hence, the choice of solvent for
ORD and CD measurements is important.

Hexane, cyclohexane, and dioxane are commonly used for ORD and CD studies. Moreover,
methanol which is transparent to low wavelengths
is a convenient solvent for the examination of
numerous chromophores.

Methanol is also the appropriate solvent
for examination of ketal-formation of a ketone,
a study which can provide very useful information on structural and stereochemical factors in
the vicinity around the carbonyl group. The acid
ketal-study has been applied to locate a methyl
group on a carbon atom adjacent to a carbonyl
(12,255). Re-investigation of this reaction
shows that it is a dimethyl-ketal and not a hemiketal which is usually formed when a ketone such
as 5α-cholestanone ($\underline{12a}$), dissolved in methanol
solution, is treated with a trace of hydrogen
chloride (256). Moreover, the ketal formation
is a reversible reaction, the ketone ⇌ ketal
equilibrium depending on the amount of water present. The formation of ketal also depends on the
nature of the alcohol, as well as on stereochem-

111

ical factors, such as the configuration around the carbonyl group. Hence, 5α-cholestan-3-one (12a) gives 96% of the dimethyl ketal, 84% of diethyl ketal, and 25% of the corresponding di-isopropyl ketal. However, a quantitative formation of the dimethyl ketal is observed in the case of a 3-keto-5β-steroid. Its diethyl ketal is formed in 94% and the corresponding diisopropyl ketal in 43% yield. These results seem to indicate that there is less steric hindrance in the ketals of 5β-3-ketones than in those of 5α-compounds and/or that the 3-keto-group is more accessible in the 5βH-series than in the 5αH-series (256).

19-Hydroxy 3-keto-steroids can exist in the free form or as a hemiketal. As shown in Fig. III-1, the magnitude of the Cotton effect associated with the 3-keto chromophore varies with the nature of the solvent, indicative of shifts in the ketone-hemiketal equilibrium (14, 20).

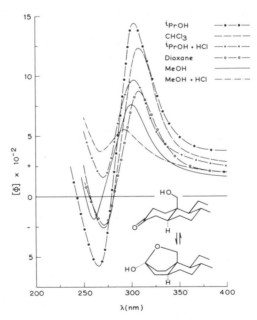

Fig. III-1.   ORD curves of 17β,19-dihydroxy-5α-androstan-3-one in different solvents (14).

The CD of a series of bicyclo-[2.2.1]-
heptanones derived from norcamphor indicates
that the Cotton effect of the ketone transition
is always more positive in a polar than a non-
polar solvent. Since these ketones are rigid,
the difference in molecular ellipticities must
be due to solvation and not to conformational
changes (15,254).
      Combination of conformational and solva-
tional equilibria are also possible. Such situ-
ations will show complex temperature variations.
Relatively widely separated CD extrema of opposite sign are usually indicative of solvation
and/or conformational equilibrium. Often, temperature-dependent and solvent-dependent ORD and
CD curves will provide information on the nature
and on the extent of both conformational and sol-
vational equilibria. In the latter case, these
data indicate solute-solvent interactions in
media such as hydrocarbons which are ordinarily
considered unlikely to participate in compound
formation (254).

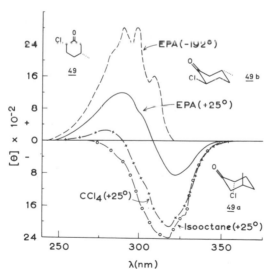

Fig. III-2. Temperature and solvent-dependent
CD curves of (+)-trans-2-chloro-5-methylcyclo-
hexanone (49) (254).

The conformational equilibrium between the diequatorial and diaxial isomers of trans-2-chloro-5-methylcyclohexanone (49) is solvent-dependent (12,15). In the non-polar solvent octane, the ketonic Cotton effect is negative, indicative of a preponderance of the conformation (49a), in which both substituents are axial. Conversely, in the polar solvent methanol, the Cotton effect is positive, in agreement with the diequatorial configuration (49b) of the substituents. In addition, this conformational equilibrium (49a) $\rightleftharpoons$ (49b) is also reflected in the temperature-dependent CD curves. As illustrated in Fig. III-2, in isooctane at 25°, the Cotton effect is negative indicative of a preponderance of the diaxial configuration (49a). In ether-isopentane-alcohol (EPA, which is a convenient solvent mixture for low-temperature studies) at -192°, the CD curve displays a positive maximum supporting the thermodynamically more stable stereochemistry (49b) (254).

5α-Androstan-11-one exhibits a positive CD curve at +25° and a negative molecular ellipticity at -192°. This unique property, attributed to a change of ring C conformation, permits to locate easily a carbonyl group in the steroid skeleton (257).

The problem of variation of Cotton effects with the dielectric constant of the solvent has been examined from a theoretical point of view (51,258). One has observed the presence of a 218 nm CD band for (S)-homo-serine-γ-lactone in water (51). The position of the band, its red shift on decreasing solvent dielectric constant, and its large anisotropy permit to assign this Cotton effect to the n-π* transition of the ester chromophore (51). Solvent and conformational effects on the dichroic properties of bridged and bicyclic lactones have been discussed in detail (.133). Dramatic effects, due to the nature of the solvents, have also been noted in the case of conjugated ketones, for which dioxane has been found to be an appropriate solvent (13,113). Similar effects have been observed with numerous other chromophores (12-15,51,133,139).

114

Often, the fine structure of the ORD and
CD curves increases by lowering the temperature,
and blue shifts are observed. In compounds with
free rotating chains, low temperature CD studies
are sometimes the only way to detect a Cotton effect (14,15,254,257).

50   50 a   50 b   50 c

The sesquiterpene nootkatone (50) may
take three possible conformations (50a), (50b),
or (50c). A CD study of (50) at various temper-
atures (from -144° in ether-isopentane-alcohol
mixture, to 133° in decalin solution) indicates
the preferred conformation of nootkatone to be
(50a) (259).

Variable-temperature CD curves of the
sesquiterpene zederone show that its conformation is rather rigid (260). Low-temperature CD
of tertiary carboxylic acids generally indicates
little conformational freedom (261). Conversely,
the CD properties of etianic acids under similar
conditions give useful information about the
preferred conformation (262).

So far, most ORD and CD measurements have
been made on liquid (solutions). However, recently the CD of (+)-3-methylcyclopentanone (6a)
vapour has been examined in the vacuum (94).
Three optically active absorption bands were observed below 200 nm, besides the usual carbonyl
$n-\pi^*$ transition around 300 nm. The CD of a crystalline solid, a mull of silicon polyether with
hexagonal crystals of L-cystine, has been reported (263). Moreover, the CD of crystalline
L-cystine and its dihydrochloride in KBr discs
has been examined in order to clear some observations made earlier and to relate the optical

properties to the conformations of disulfide groups in the crystals (264). The abnormal CD properties are the result of an exciton splitting due to the characteristic array of cystine disulfides in the crystal (264). Similarly, KCl discs have been used to establish the chirality for the propeller conformation adopted by (+)-tri-O-thymotide in the solid state. The molecule was shown to adopt the same conformation in ether solution at $-78°$ (265).

The absorption spectrum of N-[1-(p-anisyl)-2-propyl]-4-cyanopyridinium chloride, a bicyclic aromatic compound, presents a long wavelength absorption band, attributed to an intramolecular charge-transfer transition, shown to display a Cotton effect (266).

It has been mentioned (Sec. II-12) that the position of the Cotton effect of amino acids varies with the pH of the medium. Recently, it was shown that the intensity of the shorter wavelength CD band of phenyl alkyl sulfoxides depends on the degree of protonation of the SO group, and may be used to evaluate their pKa (267).

Several studies report CD Cotton effects induced in inherently symmetric chromophores by dissymmetric solvents and diastereomeric interactions of two components as solutes in an optically inactive solvent (268). The symmetric ion $[Pt\ Cl_4]^{2-}$ displays CD when dissolved in optically active 2,3-butanediol. Similar effects are observed with certain organic ketones and transition metal complexes (269). When the cation of $[Co-(NH_3)_6]^{3+}$ is precipitated as the tri $[(+)-\alpha-$bromocamphor-π-sulfonate] salt, the solid dispersed in pressed KBr discs presents clearly detectable CD in the regions of the first magnetic dipole allowed transitions of the central cobalt (III) ion (270).

Finally, the first examples of asymmetric synthesis using circularly polarized light have been reported (271).

116

References

254. A. Moscowitz, K.M. Wellman, and C. Djeras-
      si, Proc. Natl. Acad. Sci. U.S., 50, 799
      (1963); C. Djerassi, Proc. Chem. Soc., 314
      (1964); K.M. Wellman, P.H.A. Laur, W.S.
      Briggs, A. Moscowitz, and C. Djerassi, J.
      Amer. Chem. Soc., 87, 66 (1965); O.E. Wei-
      gang, J. Chem. Phys., 43, 3609 (1965); C.
      Coulombeau and A. Rassat, Bull. Soc. Chim.
      France, 2673 (1963); 3752 (1966); D.N.
      Kirk, W. Klyne, and S.R. Wallis, J. Chem.
      Soc. (C), 350 (1970).
255. C. Djerassi, L.A. Mitscher, and B.J. Mits-
      cher, J. Amer. Chem. Soc., 81, 947 (1959).
256. L.H. Zalkow, R. Hale, K. French, and P.
      Crabbé, Tetrahedron, 26, 4947 (1970).
257. K.M. Wellman, E. Bunnenberg, and C. Djeras-
      si, J. Amer. Chem. Soc., 85, 1870 (1963);
      G. Snatzke, Proceed. Roy. Soc. A, 297, 43
      (1967); Angew. Chem. Intern. Edit., 7, 14
      (1968); L. Velluz and M. Legrand, Compt.
      rend., 265, 663 (1967).
258. K. Kuriyama, T. Iwata, M. Moriyama, M.
      Ishikawa, H. Minato, and K. Takeda, J.
      Chem. Soc. (C), 420 (1967).
259. T. Ishida, T. Suga, and T. Matsuura,
      Experientia, 26, 934 (1970).
260. H. Hikino, K. Tori, I. Horibe, and K. Kuri-
      yama, J. Chem. Soc. (C), 688 (1971).
261. W.P. Mose and P.M. Scopes, J. Chem. Soc.
      (C), 1572 (1971).
262. W.P. Mose and P.M. Scopes, J. Chem. Soc.
      (C), 2417 (1971).
263. P.C. Kahn and S. Beychok, J. Amer. Chem.
      Soc., 90, 4168 (1968).
264. N. Ito and T. Takagi, Biochim. Biophys.
      Acta, 221, 430 (1970).
265. A.P. Downing, W.D. Ollis, I.O. Sutherland,
      J. Mason, and S.F. Mason, Chem. Comm., 329
      (1968).
266. A.J. de Gee, J.W. Verhoeven, I.P. Dirkx,
      and Th.J. de Boer, Tetrahedron, 25, 3407
      (1969).

267. U. Quintily and G. Scorrano, Chem. Comm.,
260 (1971).
268. K. Noack, Helv. Chim. Acta, 52, 2501
(1969); E. Axelrod, G. Barth, and E. Bunnenberg, Tetrahedron Letters, 5031 (1969);
F.A.L. Anet, L.M. Sweeting, T.A. Whitney,
and D.J. Cram, Tetrahedron Letters, 2617
(1968).
269. B. Bosnich, J. Amer. Chem. Soc., 88, 2606
(1966), 89, 6143 (1967); B. Bosnich and
D.W. Watts, J. Amer. Chem. Soc., 90, 6228
(1968).
270. B. Bosnich, J.M.B. Harrowfield, J. Amer.
Chem. Soc., 93, 4086 (1971).
271. A. Moradpour, J.F. Nicoud, G. Balavoine,
H. Kagan, and G. Tsoucaris, J. Amer. Chem.
Soc., 93, 2353 (1971); H. Kagan, A. Moradpour, J.F. Nicoud, G. Balavoine, R.H.
Martin, and J.P. Cosyn, Tetrahedron Letters, 2479 (1971), and references cited
therein.

IV. AMIDES, PEPTIDES, NUCLEOSIDES, NUCLEOTIDES, PIGMENTS, AND PORPHYRINS

IV-1. Amides, small peptides, diketopiperazines.

One common feature to numerous substances belonging to these series is the peptide moiety, which is optically active in a dissymmetric surrounding (33,34,272,273). The rotatory strength changes sign when a given perturbent is moved from one side of the peptide to the other (44,57). The detailed theoretical and experimental information of the peptide $n-\pi^*$ transition does not appear to be directly transferable to the transitions of the ester chromophore, because an α-amino group at exactly the same spatial position in the lactam imparts a negative rotatory power to the cyclic amide band around 215 nm, and in the lactone a positive optical activity to the cyclic ester transition at about the same wavelength (51,133). In the peptide unit the electronic orbitals involved in the $n-\pi^*$ transition have a higher symmetry than the group itself. The n orbital of the C-O group has a nodal surface perpendicular to the plane of the peptide group. This surface is planar in symmetrical ketones, but in peptides the vertical surface is not planar because of the horizontal distortion of the nonbonding electrons of the carbonyl group of the peptide moiety. Calculations and experiments show that this surface plays the same role as a true symmetry plane, so that the resultant rule for the peptide group is a quadrant rule, shown in Fig. IV-1 (44). Besides the $n-\pi^*$ band always observed at ca. 215 nm, the amide chromophore presents another Cotton effect about 200 nm (34,272,273).

A theoretical study of the rotational strength of the peptide transitions has appeared (57). One has shown that the anomalous behavior of dimethylamides of aldonic acids is due to a bathochromic and hyperchromic shift of the $\pi-\pi^*$ band of their amide bond (274).

In dipeptides in which the achiral glycine is either the C- or the N-terminal amino acid, a positive CD curve is observed which is much more intense than in the free amino acids. An inversion of the sign of the Cotton effect is observed around 195 nm in the case of glycyl amino acids. This transition is attributed to a $\pi-\pi^*$ band of the amide group (273). These vicinal effects, attributed to conformational changes, are discussed in some detail in Sec. V-1, (see also Appendix, Sec. V-1).

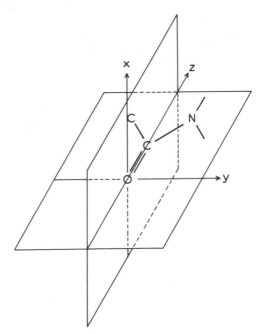

Schellman, Accounts Chem. Res. <u>1</u>, 144 (1968).

Fig. IV-1. The quadrant rule for the peptide chromophore.

The diketopiperazine chromophore, which can be considered as a cyclopeptide, exhibits various Cotton effects in the 190–230 nm range, characteristic of those of an α-helix (30,33,34, 44,133,159,239,275). In diketopiperazines formed from two different amino acids, one seems to predominate according to the polarizability (tyr(me) > tyr > phe > leu > lys) (275). In addition, the magnitude of the CD in the region of the ^1L_b-band of the aromatic chromophore of tyr-tyr-diketopiperazines, is several times larger than in linear tyr-tyr-dipeptides (276). Diketopiperazines are used as a model system to evaluate the factors determining the shapes and intensities of the near ultraviolet CD bands of the tyrosyl and tryptophanyl moieties in proteins. Cooling of the solution reveals fine structure CD bands in all of the diketopiperazines examined. Studies with c-gly-L-tyr, c-L-val-L-tyr, and c-L-phe-L-tyr confirm that the tyrosyl ^1L_b CD spectrum normally has about the same shape as the absorption spectrum. However, the CD spectra of c-L-tyr-L-tyr, are somewhat distorted, because of a small exciton CD contribution superimposed on the normal tyrosyl CD spectrum (277). The shapes of the tryptophanyl CD bands cannot be determined as precisely due to overlap of the ^1L_a and ^1L_b electronic bands. Nevertheless, the relative heights of the two major ^1L_b bands are similar in the CD spectra of c-gly-L-trp, c-L-phe-L-trp, c-L-val-L-trp, and c-D-val-L-trp. In the c-L-trp-L-trp CD spectra, however, a different ratio of ^1L_b intensities is observed, which suggests that c-L-trp-L-trp may also have a small exciton CD contribution. The tyrosyl and tryptophanyl ^1L_b fine structure CD bands apparent at low temperature can be identified in the same diketopiperazine when these bands are much more intense than the ^1L_a tryptophanyl bands, as is the case for c-L-trp-L-tyr. The identification is not as feasible when the

^1L_b intensities are low, as occurs in c-D-trp-L-tyr (277). The CD intensities are enhanced greatly in the diketopiperazines having two aromatic residues with the L configuration. This enhancement seems to result from coupling of the ^1L_b electronic transition in either a tyrosyl or tryptophanyl moiety with the far UV transitions in the second aromatic chain. Conformational equilibria were examined by cooling the diketopiperazines. The increase in CD intensity upon cooling is much less for the diketopiperazines than for the noncyclic, monomeric tyrosine and tryptophan derivatives. This finding confirms that the diketopiperazines have fewer conformers than do the noncyclic derivatives. For diketopiperazines containing only a single aromatic residue, the conformer with the aromatic chain folded over the diketopiperazine ring is dominant even at room temperature. In diketopiperazines having two aromatic residues with the L configuration, the most stable conformer has both aromatic chains sharing the space over the diketopiperazine ring (277).

The chiroptical properties of several cyclic hexapeptides have appeared. On the one hand, the CD curves of a series of cyclohexaalanyls, in the "pleated sheet" conformation, are characterized by weak $n-\pi^*$ Cotton effects around 220 nm, and two intense Cotton effects of opposite sign at ca. 205-180 nm, attributed to the split $\pi-\pi^*$ transition of the amide functions (278). On the other hand, the CD properties of several cyclic hexapeptides of glycine, leucine, tyrosine and histidine in neutral solution, indicate that they contain two transannular hydrogen bonds. These structures, which are fairly rigid, present two Cotton effects in the 220 nm and 195 nm region, attributed to the amide $n-\pi^*$ and $\pi-\pi^*$ bands, respectively (279). Several studies have been devoted to various peptide antibiotics (280).

IV-2. <u>Nucleosides, nucleotides</u>.

Nucleoproteins are found in every living cell and are made up of proteins combined with nucleic acids, which are natural polymers (Sec. V-1). The study of the primary and secondary structures of nucleic acids is fundamental, for they play a vital role in heredity.

Nucleic acids resemble proteins because they are constituted by a long chain, to which various groups are attached. By their nature and sequence these groups characterize each individual nucleic acid.

Where the backbone of the protein molecule is a polyamide chain, the polypeptide, the backbone of the nucleic acid molecule is a polyester chain, called a polynucleotide chain. The ester is derived from phosphoric acid and sugar moeity. One of a number of heterocyclic bases is attached to C-1 of each sugar through a β-linkage. A base-sugar unit is called a nucleoside. A nucleotide is a base-sugar-phosphoric acid unit.

In the group of nucleic acids known as ribonucleic acids (RNA), the sugar is D-ribose. In deoxyribonucleic acids (DNA), the sugar is D-2-deoxyribose. The bases found in DNA are adenine and guanine, which contain the purine cyclic system, and cytosine, thymine and 5-methylcytosine, which contain the pyrimidine ring. RNA contains adenine, guanine, cytosine, and uracyl. The proportions of these bases and the sequence in which they follow each other along the polynucleotide chain differ from one kind of nucleic acid to another: this is their primary structure. Their helical conformation or random coil is their secondary structure (see Sec. V-1).

Pyrimidine-riboside (51) and purine-2-deoxyriboside (52) are representative molecules belonging to this important class of natural products.

51   52

The heterocyclic systems which form the nucleosides are achiral and only become optically active in a dissymmetric surrounding. It has been shown that the electronic spectra of pyrimidines and purines can be assimilated to those of the benzene bands. Moreover, rather strong Cotton effects are observed between 200 and 300 nm (13,148,154,159,281,282).

Theoretical treatments of these chromophores have appeared, which show the π-π^* nature of the absorption spectra of the ribonucleotides in the 190–300 nm range (154,283). A method of calculating rotational strengths by a bond-bond coupled oscillatory theory, particularly in the case of the cyclonucleosides, suggests that the coupled oscillator theory accounts for most of the observed optical activity in the pyrimidine nucleosides (56). CD, one of the various experimental approaches to study nucleoside glycosidic conformation, has been used recently to examine the conformation of cytidine 2',3'-isopropylidenecytidine, uridine, and 2',3'-isopropylideneuridine in water and organic solvents. Complex concentration-dependent CD spectra have been obtained with isopropylidenecytidine and isopropylideneuridine (284). In addition, the CD data obtained on numerous pyrimidine nucleosides have allowed to study the furanose conformation as a function of the optical activity (282), (see also Appendix, Sec. IV).

Numerous accounts are devoted to the study of the chiroptical properties of these biologically important entities (159,282,285) (see also Sec. V-1). The influence of certain substituents and solvents on the CD properties of a number of guanine nucleosides are reported (286). Theoretical and empirical analyses of the data suggest that the anti conformation predominates in aqueous solution, whereas the syn conformation is preferred in alcoholic solvents, at low pH in water, and when the heterocycle carries a large substituent at position 8 of the imidazole ring (286). Theoretical calculations based on the bond-bond coupled oscillator theory are in agreement with experimental data (286).

IV-3. Pigments, porphyrins, and related substances.

The optical properties of a series of hydroxyanthraquinone pigments extracted from various streptomyces have been obtained (13). The relative stereochemistry (configuration and conformation) of aglycones of antibiotics, rhodomycinones, isorhodomycinones, and pyrromycinones are deduced from their similarly intense CD curves between 260 and 380 nm (13,161). In addition, various reports have appeared on the assignment of stereochemistry to representative members of the tetracycline group of antibiotics (161).

The porphyrins form an important class of natural substances which include chlorophyll, vitamin B_{12}, and related compounds. The tetrapyrrole nucleus present in many of these substances gives rise to complex UV spectra, indicative of numerous electronic transitions. ORD and CD measurements have been performed on various biologically active metalloporphyrins (287, 288) and chlorophyll (289). An extensive study of chlorins, which are optically active 7,8-dihydro-porphyrins, has allowed to establish empirical correlations between the molecular structures and their chiroptical properties (290). A detailed examination of the CD properties of cobalamin derivatives, specially cyanocobalamin (vitamin B_{12}) has permitted to analyze the various transitions associated with these organometallic systems (13,291).

Various accounts have appeared on the chiroptical properties of bile pigments, like stercobilin (292) and urobilins (293). Measurements of the temperature-dependent CD of l-stercobilin and d-urobilin show that the conformations of these compounds change with the temperature. The conformational changes depend on the hydrogen bonding characteristics of the solvent. The helical conformation of the dipyrrylmethene chromophore is reversed on lowering the temperature in methanol-glycerol solution, whereas in chloroform solution, reversal does not occur (293).

An interesting study reports the induced optical activity of bilirubin in the presence of sodium deoxycholate. Extrinsic Cotton effects are observed at ca. 410 and 460 nm. The sign and the magnitude of these Cotton effects depend upon the extent of association of the deoxycholate, the pH, and probably upon the ionic strength of the medium (294).

Other fundamental aspects on such chromophores, charge-transfer and helical conformation of large biomolecules (polypeptides, polynucleotides, nucleic acids, etc.) are commented upon in the following chapters.

References

272.   J.A. Schellman and P. Oriel, J. Chem. Phys., 37, 2114 (1962).

273.   M. Legrand and R. Viennet, Compt. rend., 262, 943 (1966); D.R. Dunstan and P.M. Scopes, J. Chem. Soc. (C), 1585 (1968); T. Watanabe, T. Ina, K. Ogawa, T. Matsumoto, S. Sawa, and S. Ono, Bull. Chem. Soc. Japan, 43, 3939 (1970).

274.   K. Kefurt, Z. Kefurtova, J. Nemec, J. Jary, I. Fric, and K. Bláha, Coll. Czechosl. Chem. Comm., 36, 124 (1971).

275.   D. Balasubramanian and D.B. Wetlaufer, J. Amer. Chem. Soc., 88, 3449 (1966); K. Bláha and I. Fric, Proc. Pept. Symp., 40 (1968); I.Z. Siemion, Ann., 748, 88 (1971).

276.   H. Edelhoch, R.E. Lippoldt, and M. Wilchek, J. Biol. Chem., 243, 4799 (1968).

277.   E.H. Strickland, M. Wilchek, J. Horwitz, and C. Billups, J. Biol. Chem., 245, 4168 (1970).

278.   V.T. Ivanov, V.V. Shilin, G.A. Kogan, E.N. Meshcheryakova, L.B. Senyavina, E.S. Efremov, and Y.A. Ovchinnikov, Tetrahedron Letters, 2841 (1971).

279.   St.M. Ziegler and C.A. Bush, Biochem.,
        10, 1330 (1971).
280.   S. Lee, R. Ohkawa, and N. Izumiya, Bull.
        Chem. Soc. Japan, 44, 158 (1971); S.
        Makisumi, S. Matsuura, M. Waki, and N.
        Izumiya, Bull. Chem. Soc. Japan, 44, 210
        (1971), and references cited therein.
281.   L.B. Clark and I. Tinoco, J. Amer. Chem.
        Soc., 87, 11 (1965); K.H. Scheit, 5th In-
        tern. Chem. Symp. Nat. Prod. (IUPAC),
        London (1968).
282.   I. Tinoco and Ch. R. Cantor in Methods of
        Biochemical Analysis, D. Glick (edit.),
        Vol. 18, p. 81, J. Wiley and Sons, New
        York (1970).
283.   D.W. Miles, M.J. Robins, R.K. Robins, S.
        F. Hahn, and H. Eyring, J. Phys. Chem.,
        72, 1483 (1968); D.W. Miles, W.H. Inskeep,
        M.J. Robins, M.W. Winkley, R.K. Robins,
        and H. Eyring, J. Amer. Chem. Soc., 92,
        3872 (1970).
284.   Ph. A. Hart and J.P. Davis, J. Amer. Chem.
        Soc., 93, 753 (1971).
285.   G.T. Rogers and T.L.V. Ulbricht, Biochem.
        Biophys. Res. Comm., 39, 414, 419 (1970);
        K.G. Wagner and K. Wulff, Biochem. Bio-
        phys. Res. Comm., 41, 813 (1970); K.
        Blaha, I. Fric, Z. Bezpalova, and O.
        Kaurov, Coll. Czech. Chem. Comm., 35,
        3557 (1970); R. Fecher, K.H. Boswell, J.
        J. Wittick, and T.Y. Shen, J. Amer. Chem.
        Soc., 92, 1400 (1970); M. Ikehara, S.
        Uesugi, and M. Yasumoto, J. Amer. Chem.
        Soc., 92, 4735 (1970)) T. Kunieda and B.
        Witkop, J. Amer. Chem. Soc., 91, 7751
        (1969); L.N. Nikolenko, W.N. Nesawibatko,
        A.F. Usatiy, and M.N. Semjenowa, Tetra-
        hedron Letters, 5193 (1970); M. Ikehara,
        M. Kaneko, and R. Okano, Tetrahedron, 26,
        5675 (1970); M. Ikehara, M. Kaneko, and
        M. Sagai, Tetrahedron, 26, 5757 (1970);
        Y.J.I'Haya and T. Nakamura, Bull. Chem.
        Soc. Japan, 44, 951 (1971); T. Kunieda
        and B. Witkop, J. Amer. Chem. Soc., 93,
        3478, 3493 (1971).

286. D.W. Miles, L.B. Townsend, M.J. Robins, R.K. Robins, W.H. Inskeep, and H. Eyring, J. Amer. Chem. Soc., 93, 1600 (1971).

287. S. Kirschner, Coordination Chemistry, Plenum Press, New York (1969).

288. G.L. Eichhorn, Tetrahedron, 13, 208 (1961).

289. B. Ke and R.B. Miller, Naturwiss., 51, 436 (1964).

290. H. Wolf, Ann. Chem., 695, 98 (1966), and subsequent papers by this author; see also Chap. 20 in ref. 15; H. Wolf and H. Scheer, Ann. Chem., 745, 87 (1971).

291. L. Velluz, M. Legrand, and R. Viennet, Compt. rend., 255, 15 (1962); M. Legrand and R. Viennet, Bull. Soc. Chim. France, 1435 (1962).

292. H. Plieninger and J. Ruppert, Ann. Chem., 736, 43 (1970).

293. C.H. Gray, P.M. Jones, W. Klyne, and D.C. Nicholson, Nature, 184, 41 (1959); A. Moscowitz, W.C. Krueger, I.T. Kay, G. Skewes, and S. Bruckenstein, Proc. Natl. Acad. Sci. U.S., 52, 1190 (1964); D.A. Lightner, E.L. Docks, J. Horwitz, and A. Moscowitz, Proc. Natl. Acad. Sci. U.S., 67, 1361 (1970); H. Plieninger, K. Ehl, and A. Tapia, Ann. Chem., 736, 62 (1970).

294. J.H. Perrin and M. Wilsey, Chem. Comm., 769 (1971).

V. OPTICALLY ACTIVE POLYMERS

At the beginning of this Century, some
natural substances, later recognized to be high
polymers, were shown to exhibit optical activity.
However, the unsatisfactory purification techniques available at that time made that their optical properties were not investigated further.
Polarimetry was then used almost exclusively for
structural and stereochemical study of small molecules.
During the last twenty years, not only
did new improvements occur in the field of in-
strumentation in ORD and CD, but biopolymers of
high purity also became available. Thus, a considerable attention has been devoted to the examination of the chiroptical properties of natural polymers. In addition a substantial number
of optically active synthetic high polymers have
been prepared and their optical properties investigated.

V-1.   <u>Naturally occurring polymers</u>.

Spectroscopic methods and particularly
ORD and CD have undoubtedly played an important
part in the study of biomolecules. Since several
books and review articles are now available on
protein conformation, nucleoproteins, ribosomes,
viruses, lipoproteins, membranes, and other
macromolecules (12-15,159,282,295,296), only
salient points and some recent results will be
mentioned here. Moreover, a comprehensive survey
of the current status of theoretical and experimental studies of conformations of polypeptides
has appeared (297).
All naturally occurring biopolymers, formed

of carbohydrates or amino acid units, like poly-
saccharides, proteins, and polypeptides, polynucleotides and enzymes (including cellulose,
dextran, gelatin, etc.) exhibit optical activity
(12-15). The chiroptical properties depend on
both their primary structure (i.e., the specific
chemical composition) and their secondary structure (i.e., the helix or random coil). Even if
the structural information that they are able to
deliver is of a low order, their place in protein
chemistry is secure. Thus, ORD and CD techniques are used routinely to follow isolation
procedures of biomolecules, to check their purity, their storage conditions, to study reduction
reactions, denaturation and degradation, etc.
Moreover, the chiroptical techniques have been
applied to such studies as modification of the
nature of the solvent, degree of solvation, variations of the pH of the medium, modifications of
the temperature, etc.

The discovery of the anomalous dispersion
of α-helical polypeptides establishes conformational rotations due to the helical structure
(30,33,34,295). Moreover, native proteins in
general are known to exhibit much less negative
rotations than do denatured proteins, so that it
was suggested that such changes in rotations were
associated with loss of helical structures. An
equation explaining the ORD properties of α-helical polypeptides has been used as the basis for
the estimation of the α-helix content of many
types of synthetic polypeptides and proteins. A
discussion of this problem from a theoretical
point of view assumes exciton coupling and shows
that strong Cotton effects of opposite signs
(couplet) should originate from each strong elec-
tronic transitions such as the $\pi^{\circ} \longrightarrow \pi$ transition
at 190 nm, which have parallel and perpendicular
polarization with respect to the axis of the α-
helix (30,298). It was shown later that for an
infinitively long helix they cause the appearance of another couplet. This refined exciton
treatment predicts, therefore, four bands for
each strong absorption. For the α-helix they are

expected to occur at 185, 189, and 193 nm. In
addition, as indicated in Sec. IV-1, the n-π*
transition of the peptide bond is also predicted
to be optically active near 215 nm (44,272,273).
Presently available instruments do not allow to
resolve these five bands completely, specially
below 190 nm. In spite of the more complex results of the refined theory, the original treatment by Moffitt describes satisfactorily the
chiroptical behaviour of the α-helix, confirmed
by polarization measurements (12-15). This is
illustrated experimentally by CD studies of poly-
L-glutamic acid (272,273), which indicate the α-
helix to display complex Cotton effect curves at
ca. 220 nm, corresponding to the n-π* transition
of the amide chromophore and a 200 nm band, due
to its π-π* transition (Sec. IV-1). This observation agrees with the studies mentioned above,
indicating that the simple transition of the amide chromophore should appear as a double band,
because of the presence of this chromophore in
an helical structure. When the polypeptide or
the protein is denatured, this complex system
disappears: one observes only the weak n-
CD maximum and a simple π-π* transition. Hence,
the characteristic CD curve, typical of α-helix,
permits to measure easily the chirality in proteins.

It should be mentioned however, that similar complex CD curves have been observed with
some simple amides, like methylpyrrolidone (299),
indicating that an S-type CD curve does not necessarily reflect an helicoidal conformation of
the chromophore.

In addition, a careful study of various
proteins has allowed to detect the β form presented by some of them (300). In this form instead of being distributed in space along an
helix, the chromophores are located in a plane.
The CD curves of such proteins also present an S
shape, but the magnitude of the Cotton effects is
less than in the α-helix conformation. For example, the ORD and CD of phytochrome in the P_R and
P_{FR} forms were determined between 200 and 500 nm.

The CD spectra below 240 nm correspond closely with that assigned to the β-chain configuration. If the protein is considered to be a mixture of α-helix and random coil, the ellipticity at 220 nm would correspond to an α-helix content of 14% (301).

The theoretical calculation of the helix senses of a number of homopolyamino acids has been reported (297). The predicted existence of the right-handed α-helical form of poly-L-valine was verified by incorporating poly-L-valine into a block copolymer, between two blocks of poly-DL-lysine. ORD and CD showed that around 50% of the short valine block of $(DL-lysine\ hydrochloride)_{18}-(L-valine)_{15}-(DL-lysine\ hydrochloride)_{16}-glycine$ was found to be in the right-handed α-helical conformation in aqueous methanol solution. Hence, as predicted, there is no steric hindrance preventing the formation of the α-helix in this polyamino acid. The predicted senses of the α-helical forms of the o- and m-chlorobenzyl esters of poly-L-aspartic acid were checked by ORD and CD studies. As predicted, these polymers draw left-handed α-helices, in contrast to the para-isomer which forms a right-handed α-helix (297).

The conformational study of nucleoproteins is more difficult than the work on simple proteins, for the nucleic acid component itself is optically active (296,302,303). The optical activity of nucleic acids is caused by both the dissymmetry in each of the many pentose residues, as well as by the ordered conformation of the polynucleotide chain. In spite of the fact that the chiroptical properties of nucleic acids are complicate, they allow to distinguish between simple or complex helices and to show that the pH and temperature are important factors acting on their conformation. The recently described measurements of CD and UV spectra of DNA oriented by flow provide new support for the theory of polynucleotide optical activity advanced earlier (304,305).

The properties associated with the active disulfide transitions (Sec. II-21), as well as

the CD of some specific proteins such as myoglobin, haemoglobin, insulin, ribonuclease,
serum albumin, and lysozyme have been reported
(159,282,295,296,302). In addition, the chiroptical methods have been used to provide information about the structure of nucleohistones,
stabilization of ribonucleic acids with natural
or synthetic polybases, and action of urea and
sodium dodecylsulfate on the structure of oval-
bumine, etc. Moreover, recent studies have
shown that in globular proteins, Cotton effects
often of considerable magnitude occur in the
near UV absorption bands of tyrosine and tryptophan. An account on the optical activity of
tryptophan and phenylalanine derivatives and of
tyrosine, in relation particularly to ribonuclease, shows a substantial Cotton effect associated with the absorption band of its six tyrosine residues. A systematic analysis of these
effects has been attempted (306). A series of
simple derivatives examined in glassy solvents
at liquid nitrogen temperature show fine-structure in both UV and CD, which makes it possible
to analyze the vibrational composition of the
bands. The phenolic chromophore contains two
transitions in the near UV. The corresponding
vibrational progressions, one strong and one
weak, have been examined. Their positions are
very solvent-sensitive, and it is therefore to
be expected that in ribonuclease, which has
three buried and three exposed tyrosine moieties,
there will be progressions arising from both
classes if both show enhanced optical activity.
At low temperature fine-structure appears, and
with the aid of a curve-resolver, bands repre-
senting the first members of three progressions
can be discerned, two from internal and one from
the external, solvent-perturbed, residues. A
large disulfide contribution extending to long
wavelengths is also evident. Thus it is in principle possible to distinguish not only tyrosine
from tryptophan components, but also internal
from external ones, and the possibility arises of
observing events around individual aromatic residues in globular proteins (306).

The optical properties of poly-L-tyrosine are very different from those of simple polypeptides. Comparison of calculated and experimental CD curves indicate that poly-L-tyrosine forms a right-handed helix (58). One has also shown that the chiroptical properties of formophenolic polycondensates of N-tosyl L-tyrosine change with the nature of the solvent and the pH of the medium (307).

Some applications of the chiroptical techniques in following changes in structure have been reported. Conjugated proteins, such as those containing haem, show complex systems of Cotton effects in the absorption region of the prosthetic groups. The Cotton effects of the cytochrome C_3 of three related sulfate-reducing bacteria have been described (308). In spite of their low molecular weight, these proteins are reported to carry three haem groups each. They have very large Cotton effects, showing that in spite of the considerable differences in amino acid composition the three proteins are effectively identical in terms of the haem environment. On acid denaturation, there is a sharp diminution in the Cotton effects, and this can be used to follow the denaturation with great precision.

Measurements of the ORD and CD of various membranes and membrane systems have been reported (309). The interpretation proved difficult, because of the macroscopic nature of the material. The effects of differential scattering of left and right-circularly polarized light have been analyzed, and it was shown that it can in principle account for much of the distorted shape of the peptide Cotton effects observed in these systems (309). In spite of this complication, however, it is sometimes possible to extract useful information from the CD of membranes. For example, it has been found that the peptide Cotton effects, and therefore the protein conformation, do not change on treatment with phospholipase, which leads to the release of most of the total phospholipid (310). Further-

more, the digestion is accompanied by the emer-
gence of a series of resonances in the NMR spectrum, not evident in the intact membrane, and
corresponding to the spectrum of extracted
lipids in solution. Conversely, when membranes
are heated, the breakdown of the protein structure can be followed by the change in CD, and
this is associated with the appearance of the
NMR spectrum of unfolded protein chains, but not
of the methylene resonances of the fatty acid
lipid chains, which evidently remain essentially
immobile. Hence, it seems that the disordering
of the proteins and of the lipids are independent
and unrelated processes. It is inferred that
the proteins are directly associated with only the
minor fraction of phospholipids that are not de-
stroyed by phospholipase, and are distributed in
self-contained packets in a lipid bilayer matrix
(310).

The ORD and CD techniques have also been
used to study charge-transfer absorption bands
associated with intra- and intermolecular elec-
tron-donor-acceptor-complexes in chiral molecules (311).

Addition of optically inactive dyes to
helical polypeptides results in a Cotton effect
in the visible wavelength range. Dye-polymer
adducts exhibit induced Cotton effects, attributed to oriented interactions of the dye molecule with the macromolecular helix (12,14,15).
These Cotton effects disappear by destruction of
the helical conformation when the pH of the solution is modified (312,313). For example, such
induced Cotton effects have been observed with
DNA-acridine orange, RNA-proflavin, DNA-amino-
acridine, as well as amylose with different dyes
(313).

An interesting account describes the Cotton effect induced in an optically inactive aromatic amine added to RNA or to DNA (314). The
molecule displays a positive CD maximum at about
360 nm when added to RNA and a negative maximum
when added to DNA. These results are reminiscent of the chiroptical properties associated
with charge-transfer transitions and observed

for intra- and intermolecular electron-donor-
acceptor-complexes of amino acids (Sec. II-12
and VI) and peptides (311) and suggest a potential method to study helix topography. Moreover, CD experiments indicate that lysergic acid
diethylamide (LSD) interacts directly with puri-
fied calf thymus DNA, probably the intercalation
causing conformational changes in the DNA (315).
CD studies along with X-ray diffraction indicate
that poly d(1-C), poly d(1-C), an unusual double-
helical DNA, exists in a new polynucleotide configuration, an eight-fold helix, possibly left-
handed (316).

Mild treatment of a variety of proteins
with diazotized p-arsanilic acid, modifying only
a fraction of the total number of the potential-
ly reactive residues present, generates azo
proteins with CD bands above 300 nm (317). The
interaction of ribonuclease St with guanosine
3'-monophosphate, a competitive inhibitor for
the enzyme, has also been studied by means of CD
(318). Specific complexes between oligoribonu-
cleotides have also been investigated by CD
(319).

In addition, several recent publications
are devoted to such topics as CD studies of DNA
complexes with arginine-rich histone IV (320),
CD of native and illuminated bovine visual pig-
ment (321), ORD properties of nucleic acid complexes with the oligopeptide antibiotics dista-
mycin A and netropsin (322), etc. (323).

A report mentions a new experimental method providing both the structural information obtained from ORD experiments and information on
the molecular geometry from evaluation of the
relaxion time. Applications for biopolymer char-
acterization are mentioned (324).

Finally, an important study is devoted to
the origin of the heme Cotton effects in myoglobin and hemoglobin (325). The rotational
strengths of the heme $\pi-\pi^*$ transitions in these
two proteins were calculated. Heme Cotton effects of mutant hemoglobins and other heme
proteins are discussed, based on the mechanism
identified in myoglobin and hemoglobin (325).

136

Briefly, the most important results of the ORD and CD studies with biopolymers can be summarized as follows. The far UV Cotton effects support the right-handed α-helix and the extended β-structures are the common conformations in globular and fibrous proteins. Several proteins present either rigid or flexible polypeptide chains in which no repeating orders could be observed. The chiroptical methods are helpful in showing and confirming the contention that the secondary and tertiary structures are determined by the primary structure (amino acid composition and sequence). The ORD and CD reports of glycoproteins show that the carbohydrate constituents have an adverse effect on the formation and stability of α-helices, perhaps because of the hydrophylic nature of the carbohydrate. Studies of lipoproteins indicate that in some cases the lipid stabilizes the helices. Furthermore, some of the lipid components may contribute to some extend to the modification of the Cotton effects. ORD and CD studies are of primary help to study enzyme activity mechanisms, such as by disclosing conformational changes in coenzyme binding, in substrate binding and in interactions with inhibitors. Investigations of immunoglobulins provide information about their conformation and about the role of conformation in antibody specificity. The chiroptical methods are contributing substantially to structural studies of the fibrous structural proteins, such as myosins, keratins, silks and collagens. In addition, the conformation of histones and nucleoproteins has been elucidated and the ability of the various histone fractions to assume helical conformation has been shown to depend on the proline content. Finally, ORD and CD studies are very useful to comparative biochemistry and taxonomy of proteins and nucleic acids (296).

Since life processes depend crucially on electron interactions between organic molecules and metal ions, all attempts to understand better the transitions and stereochemistry of ligands, as well as polypeptides and nucleic acids constitute important steps forward in scientific knowledge.

V-2.   Synthetic high polymers.

The discovery of polymerization catalysts capable of producing polymers with various stereoregularity, raised the problem of the relationship between conformation of stereoregular macromolecules in the crystalline state and in the liquid state or in solution, as well as between stereoregularity and conformation (326). A theoretical approach for the interpretation of optical activity in stereoregular polymers has appeared (326). It is based on the fundamental concepts developed with biopolymers (30,33,34, 305). The empirical method of calculation of the rotatory power (84,334) has also provided satisfactory results with some synthetic polymers (326).

The chiroptical properties of some polyhydrocarbons, polyalkenylethers, polyacrylic derivatives, and polyaldehydes have been obtained (133,326-328). One has shown that there is a relationship between the sign of the Cotton effects and the helical conformations of poly-α-olefins. Interesting phenomena have been observed with polyacrylates and polylactides. In such compounds anomalies in ORD curves have been noted, whilst such anomalies are not present in the curves of low molecular weight esters and lactones.

Since the optical activity is proportional to the content of asymmetric monomer, the reactivity ratios can be deduced from the analysis of copolymers from optically inactive and active monomers (329,330). As in biopolymers, isomerization rates, racemization and denaturation processes of optically active synthetic polymers may also be deduced from their chiroptical properties.

The mode of action of complex catalysts may be examined by ORD and CD, provided that the catalysts are labeled with asymmetric groups (331). The stereochemistry of propagation mecha-

138

nisms can also be investigated by these methods
(332). A recent account reports the change in
the rotatory direction of optically active poly
(propylene oxide) in different solvents. This
is discussed from the viewpoint of dielectric
theory in solution (333). It seems that in such
cases the shapes of the ORD curves of polymers
cannot be related to their conformation (333).
        A considerable amount of work has been
devoted to the examination of the optical properties of active polymers with asymmetric carbon
atoms in the main chain. These studies include
polymers from three-membered heterocyclic compounds, polyesters, polythiolesters, polyamides
and polymers of dienic monomers. Similarly, the
chiroptical properties of polymers with dissymmetric side chains (e.g. polyvinylethers, poly-
alkylvinylketones, polyacrylic derivatives, polyaldehydes, etc.) have also been described (326).
In most cases, useful correlations could be established between the experimental data obtained
with stereoregular synthetic polymers, in particular poly-α-olefins, and theoretical considerations (326,334).
        One of the main problems in synthetic
polymers is the determination of their chemical
structure for highly stereoregular polymers have
been obtained in relatively few cases. And it
is only when the structural problem has been
solved that optical methods can be applied to
the study of their stereochemistry. So far, the
theoretical treatment of the optical properties
of polymers has given promising results only in
these cases where strong interaction exists between chromophoric systems regularly ordered
along the polymer main chain. Such a type of interaction has only been observed in poly-α-amino-
acids. The interactions noted in the n-π* transitions of polyvinylketones, polymetacrylic
esters and polyacrylamides are rather weak and
need further research (326). It remains, however, that synthetic high polymers is another
area in which the ORD and CD techniques will show
their potential in the future, because the chi-

roptical properties will help to clarify conformational features not easily deduced from other
physical methods.

References

295. G.D. Fasman, Poly-α-Amino Acids, M. Dekker,
     Inc., New York (1967).
296. B. Jirgensons, Optical Rotatory Dispersion
     of Proteins and Other Macromolecules,
     Springer-Verlag, New York (1969).
297. H.A. Scheraga, Chem. Rev., 71, 195 (1971).
298. W. Moffitt and J.T. Yang, Proc. Natl. Acad.
     Sci. U.S., 42, 596 (1956); W. Moffitt,
     Proc. Natl. Acad. Sci. U. S., 42, 736
     (1956).
299. D.W. Urry, J. Phys. Chem., 72, 3035 (1968).
300. P.K. Sarkar and P. Doty, Proc. Natl. Acad.
     Sci. U. S., 55, 981 (1966).
301. G.R. Anderson, E.L. Jenner, and F.E. Mum-
     ford, Biochim. Biophys. Acta, 221, 69
     (1970).
302. Sh. Beychok in Poly-α-Amino Acids, G.D.
     Fasman (edit.), Chap. 7, p. 293, M. Dekker,
     Inc., New York (1967).
303. J. Brahms and W.F.H. Mommaerts, J. Molec.
     Biol., 10, 73 (1964); J. Brahms, J. Molec.
     Biol., 11, 785 (1965); K.E. Van Holde, J.
     Brahms, and A.M. Michelson, J. Molec. Biol.,
     12, 726 (1965); 15, 467 (1966); J. Brahms,
     J.C. Maurizot, and A.M. Michelson, J.
     Molec. Biol., 25, 465 (1967).
304. S.Y. Wooley and G. Holzwarth, J. Amer.
     Chem. Soc., 93, 4066 (1971).
305. I. Tinoco, J. Chim. Phys. Physicochim.
     Biol., 65, 91 (1968); W.C. Johnson and I.
     Tinoco, Biopolymers, 7, 727 (1969).
306. J. Horwitz, E.H. Strickland, and C. Billups,
     J. Amer. Chem. Soc., 92, 2119 (1970).
307. M. Vert and E. Sélégny, Bull. Soc. Chim.
     France, 663 (1971).
308. H. Drucker, L.L. Campbell, and R.W. Woody,
     Biochem., 9, 1519 (1970).

309. D.W. Urry and J. Krivacic, Proc. Natl. Acad. Sci. U.S., 65, 845 (1970); C.A. Ottaway, and D.B. Wetlaufer, Arch. Biochem. Biophys., 139, 257 (1970).

310. M. Glaser, H. Simpkins, S.J. Singer, M. Sheetz, and S.I. Chan, Proc. Natl. Acad. Sci. U.S., 65, 721 (1970).

311. P. Moser, Helv. Chim. Acta, 51, 1831 (1968).

312. L. Stryer and E.R. Blout, J. Amer. Chem. Soc., 83, 1411 (1961); G. Scheibe, F. Haimerl, and W. Hoppe, Tetrahedron Letters, 3067 (1970).

313. E.R. Blout, Tetrahedron, 13, 123 (1961); D.M. Neville and D.F. Bradley, Biochim. Biophys. Acta, 50, 397 (1961); A. Blake and A.R. Peacocke, Nature, 206, 1009 (1965); R.E. Ballard, A.J. McCaffery, and S.F. Mason, Biopolymers, 4, 97 (1966); B. J. Gardner and S.F. Mason, Biopolymers, 5, 79 (1967); K. Sensse and F. Cramer, Chem. Ber., 102, 509 (1969); H.M. Bössler and R. C. Schulz, Koll. Zeitsch. und Zeitsch. Polym., 239, 578 (1970).

314. E.J. Gabbay, J. Amer. Chem. Soc., 90, 6574 (1968).

315. Th.E. Wagner, Nature, 222, 1170 (1969).

316. Y. Mitsui, R. Langridge, B.E. Shortle, Ch. R. Cantor, R.C. Grants, M. Kodama, and R. D. Wells, Nature, 228, 1166 (1970).

317. C.F. Fairclough and B.L. Vallee, Biochem., 9, 4087 (1970).

318. N. Yoshida, K. Kuriyama, T. Iwata, and H. Otsuka, Biochem. Biophys. Res. Comm., 43, 954 (1971).

319. R.B. Gennis and Ch.R. Cantor, Biochem., 9, 4714 (1970).

320. T.Y. Shih and G.D. Fasman, Biochem., 10, 1675 (1971).

321. J. Horwitz and J. Heller, Biochem., 10, 1402 (1971).

322. Ch. Zimmer and G. Luck, FEBS Letters, 10, 339 (1970).

323. G.D. Fasman, H. Hoving, and S.N. Timasheff,
     Biochem., 9, 3316 (1970); K. Ruckpaul, H.
     Rein, O. Ristau, and F. Jung, Experientia,
     26, 1079 (1970); K. Ruckpaul, H. Rein, O.
     Ristau, and F. Jung, Biochim. Biophys.
     Acta, 221, 9 (1970); E. Fujimori and J.
     Pecci, Biochim. Biophys. Acta, 221, 132
     (1970); M. Ekblad, Th.A. Bewley, and H.
     Papkoff, Biochim. Biophys. Acta, 221, 142
     (1970); D.G. Dearborn and D.B. Wetlaufer,
     Biochem. Biophys. Res. Comm., 39, 314
     (1970); K. Wulff, H. Wolf, and K.G. Wagner,
     Biochem. Biophys. Res. Comm., 39, 870
     (1970); Th.E. Wagner, Nature, 227, 65
     (1970); E. Peggion, L. Strasorier, and A.
     Cosani, J. Amer. Chem. Soc., 92, 381
     (1970); F.C. Yong and T.E. King, Biochem.
     Biophys. Res. Comm., 40, 1445 (1970); Y.A.
     Ovchinnikov, V.T. Ivanov, and I.I. Mikha-
     leva, Tetrahedron Letters, 159 (1971); M.
     W. Makinen and H. Kon, Biochem., 10, 43
     (1971); B. Pfannemüller, H. Mayerhöfer, and
     R.C. Schulz, Biopolymers, 10, 243 (1971);
     H.A. McKenzie and G.B. Ralston, Experientia,
     27, 617 (1971).
324. B.R. Jennings and E.D. Baily, Nature, 228,
     1309 (1970).
325. M.C. Hsu and R.W. Woody, J. Amer. Chem.
     Soc., 93, 3515 (1971).
326. P. Pino, F. Ciardelli, and M. Zandomeneghi,
     in Ann. Rev. Phys. Chem., 561 (1970).
327. P. Pino, Adv. Polymer Sci., 4, 393 (1965);
     P. Pino, G.P. Lorenzi, and O. Bonsignori,
     Chim. Ind. (Milan), 48, 760 (1966); P. Sal-
     vadori, L. Lardicci, and P. Pino, Tetra-
     hedron Letters, 1641 (1965); P. Salvadori,
     L. Lardicci, G. Consiglio, and P. Pino,
     Tetrahedron Letters, 5343 (1966); P. Pino,
     C. Carlini, E. Chiellini, F. Ciardelli,
     and P. Salvadori, J. Amer. Chem. Soc., 90,
     5025 (1968).

328. R.C. Schulz and E. Kaiser, Adv. Polymer Sci., 4, 236 (1965); R.C. Schulz and R.H. Jung, Makromol. Chem., 96, 295 (1966); R. Wolf and R.C. Schulz, J. Macromol Sci., A2 (4), 821 (1968); B. Pfannemüller, H. Mayer-höfer, and R.C. Schulz, Makromol. Chem., 121, 147 (1969).
329. R.C. Schulz in Encyclopaedia of Polymer Science and Technology, Vol. 9, John Wiley and Sons, Inc., New York (1968).
330. M. Goodman, A. Abe, and Y.L. Fan in Polymer Handbook, Interscience Publ., New York (1966); A. Abe, J. Amer. Chem. Soc., 92, 1136 (1970).
331. G. Natta, L. Porri, and S. Valenti, Makromol. Chem., 67, 225 (1963).
332. S. Inoue, Y. Yokota, N. Yoshida, and T. Tsuruta, Makromol. Chem., 90, 131 (1966); T. Tsuruta, S. Inoue, and Y. Yokota, Makromol. Chem., 103, 164 (1967); Y. Kumata, J. Furukawa, and T. Saegusa, Makromol. Chem., 105, 138 (1967); 81, 100 (1965).
333. Y. Kumata, J. Furukawa, and T. Fueno, Bull. Chem. Soc. Japan, 43, 3663, 3920 (1970).
334. J.H. Brewster, J. Amer. Chem. Soc., 81, 5475 (1959).

VI. METALLIC COMPLEXES

Most optically active compounds are organic molecules. However, optical activity is
not a unique feature of dissymmetric entities
formed of carbon, sulfur, nitrogen, or phosphorus
atoms, because Cotton effect curves have also
been observed in molecules of higher degree of
symmetry (15). For example, tris[dihydroxo
tetrammin cobalt(III)] cobalt(III) hexanitrate
is optically active. The bidendate ligand (53),
symbolized by A-A is an octahedral complex, namely the species shown in (54). The A's represent
the hydroxyl groupings forming a total of six
bridges between the central and the three coordinated cobalt atoms (15).

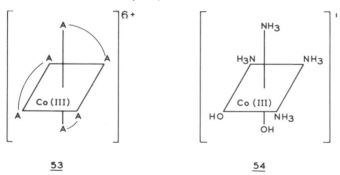

53   54

Numerous optically active inorganic substances are in fact metal-organic compounds whose
electronic patterns differ substantially from
classical organic molecules (287). In contrast
to many active organic molecules, usually the metallic complexes have to be resolved, since it
is only seldom that nature provides active com-

plexes (such as in chlorophyll or vitamin B_{12}) (288,289). In spite of this drawback, numerous metallic complexes have been examined by ORD and CD, since the chiroptical properties allow to study at the same time the optical activity as such, as well as symmetry and stereochemical features. For example, the phenomenon of isomerism due to non-planarity of chelate rings, such as in complexes of amines, can be examined by ORD and CD. In addition, Cotton effects are observed for transitions corresponding to polarization directions parallel or perpendicular to symmetry axes, mainly for $d \longrightarrow d$ transition at high wavelength (15,287,335,336).

Usually, the long-wavelength absorption band of transition metal complexes is due to an electronic transition of the magnetic-dipole type. The optical properties of several metal complexes with symmetries lower than dihedral, as well as those with three bidendate ligands, have been measured in order to assign spectroscopic transitions and to establish the absolute configuration. The origin of the optical activity in metal complexes has also been studied theoretically. The contribution played by ORD and CD has been fundamental in this field, because the sign of the rotation at a particular wavelength cannot be used to relate the configurations of various substances, since they possess several absorption bands.

Not only can compounds containing an asymmetric carbon atom be resolved into enantiomers, but this also applies to other main-group elements, such as arsenic, beryllium, boron, germanium, nitrogen, phosphorus and silicon, when they are situated at the center of a tetrahedron with four different substituents. A detailed review on the optical activity from asymmetric transition metal atoms has appeared (337). In addition, the application of the exciton theory (27) to the determination of the absolute configuration of inorganic complexes has been reported (338). The method can be applied to the class of dissymmetric coordination compounds containing

conjugated ligands typified by the three strongly coordinating bidendate ligands, o-phenanthro-
line, 2,2'-bipyridyl, and the acetylacetonate
ion (338).

Little is known about the asymmetric in-
duction exerted by an s-butyl group in an olefin
when at least one of the unsaturated carbon atoms
becomes asymmetric by complexion of the olefin
to a transition metal. A recent CD study shows
that the s-butyl asymmetric carbon atom originally present in cis- and trans-dichloro(benzylamine) (olefin) platinum(II) complexes induces
an opposite absolute configuration in the tertiary carbon atom bond to the platinum atom (339).
Furthermore, CD has helped to clarify the trans
addition reaction of a nucleophile to a platinum
(II) coordinated simple olefin (340).

Since amino acids ions form stable chelate
compounds with various metals, their configuration can be deduced from the optical properties.
A CD study of $Co[(NH_3)_5$-L-amino acid-H$]$ X_3 complexes shows that they belong to symmetry C_{4v}
(341). Nickel(II) (144,342) and copper(II) (145)
complexes of amino acids have also been investigated by CD. The data of the latter complexes
cannot be explained by any octant or quadrant
rule (vide infra). Instead, an hexadecant rule
is proposed, which accounts for the sign identity
and magnitude additivity observed in these complexes (145). For example, in a same class of
symmetry D_2, the CD curves differ according to
the nature of the ligands: bisdiamino cis-Co
$(en)_2$ L_2^{3+} complexes show a different number of
bands when L is unidendate or bidendate (343).

An octant rule for octahedral complexes of
Co(III) suggests that for classes of given symmetry, the absolute configuration can be deduced
from the sign of the Cotton effects at high wavelengths (344). The derivation of the octant sign
for a variety of structures and the possibility
to correlate the octant sign and the sign of the
Cotton effects for identified transitions within

147

certain symmetry groups are mentioned (i.e. mono-
bidentate, bis-bidentate, tris-bidentate and mul-
tibidentate complexes) (344). Moreover, a double octant rule has been proposed for planar
transition metal ion complexes (345). Recently,
sector or symmetry rules which govern the signs
and relative magnitudes of the rotatory strengths
associated with ligand-field transitions have
been proposed for metal complexes of the pseudo-
tetragonal class (346). In addition, a quadrant
rule has been suggested for the d-d transitions
of platinum(II)-olefin complexes (347).

The chiroptical properties in the visible
region of metallic complexes give information
about the stereochemistry around the central ion,
whereas charge-transfer transitions, which appear at lower wavelengths, reflect the configuration of the ring chelated on itself (348). Steric interactions in amino acid complexes are
easily detected by CD, since the sign and intensity of the Cotton effects reflect the conformation of the chelated rings (349).

Various studies are devoted to effects on
active transitions (350) and to the possible contribution of neighboring orbitals to orbitals of
the metal, in complexes of type [Co X(CN)en$_2$]X
(351).

Besides the most investigated cobalt complexes (13,146,291,345,352,353), the chiroptical
properties of numerous nickel, copper, and molybdate organo-metallic derivatives have been reported (15,74,88,90,143-146,287,335,336,354).
Among the chiroptical properties of platinum complexes (15,88), one should mention a recent investigation of the interaction between dichloro
(1,5-hexadiene) platinum(II) and (S)-α-methyl-
benzylamine (355). The addition reaction affords
a derivative containing a carbon-platinum σ-bond.
Monomeric and binuclear products are obtained and
both exhibit multiple Cotton effect CD curves
(355). A general periodic trend, related to the
ionic potential of the lanthanide(III) ions, was
noted in the ORD spectra of the lanthanide-D-(-)-
1,2-propylenediaminetetraacetato complexes (356).

The CD and UV spectra of a series of nickel (II) complexes with tetradentate Schiff bases derived from (R)-(-)propane-1,2-diamine and (R,R)-(-)-cyclohexane-1,2-diamine have been measured. The signs of the Cotton effects have been correlated with the preferred conformation of the central chelate ring produced by the stereochemical requirements of the ligands. The CD curves of these compounds, in general, reveal more band multiplicity than do the corresponding UV spectra (357).

A recent account reports the optical activity induced into the tetrachlorides of tin (IV), titanium(IV), and zirconium(IV), using d-tartaric acid and d- and l-malic acids as environment compounds (358). Examination of the CD properties indicates the formation of hexacoordinate species with the solvent (DMF) (358).

Several other studies have been devoted to the stereochemistry of complexes with arsenic, iron, palladium, chromium, ruthenium, rhodium, mercury, vanadium, etc. (353,354,359).

The present state of knowledge may be summarized as follows. Although CD in solution was first observed by Cotton in 1895, in the visible absorption region of transition metal complexes, the chiroptical properties of coordination compounds are less well-understood than these of dissymmetric organic molecules. This is due to the greater number and variety of excitation processes in metal complexes in which, in addition to the electronic transitions of the organic ligand, are added those of the metal ion and the metalligand charge-transfer excitations (360). Hence, usually, metal complexes display three types of electronic transitions which may be regarded as occurring within the d-electron manifold (d-d transitions), between the metal and the ligands (charge-transfer), and transitions which are essentially localized on the ligands (338,360). In optically active metal-organic complexes these three transitions exhibit a Cotton effect, but at present it is only the last type of transition which can be used to correlate the sign of the CD curve with the absolute

configuration (338,360). Thus, the absolute stereochemistry of a bis- or tris-chelated coordination compound containing unsaturated ligands
is deduced from the sign and the energy-order of
the major CD bands associated with the internal
ligand $\pi-\pi^*$ transitions. The sign of the Cotton effect associated with a $\pi-\pi^*$ transition
polarized along the principal rotational axis of
the complex reflects the chirality of the ligands
around the metal ion with respect to that axis,
positive for the $\Delta(C_3)$ configuration of complexes
with D_3 or C_3 symmetry or the $\Delta(C_2)$ configuration
of bis-chelate complexes with two-fold rotational
symmetry. The associated $\pi-\pi^*$ transition polarized perpendicularly to the principal rotational
axis shows a CD band of opposite sign at higher
frequency in the case of the C_2 complex, or at
lower frequency in the case of the C_3 or D_3 complex (360).

Ring-metal π-complexes, or metallocenes,
are of interest since their molecular geometry
is a challenging stereochemical problem, for
which the chiroptical methods can provide useful
information.

Monosubstituted metallocenes belong to the
point group C_s. Homoannular substitution with
a group R_2 different from the first R_1 affords
disubstituted products belonging to the point
group C_1. Such compounds are chiral and can be
resolved. Several optically active metallocenes
of known configuration have been prepared. In
some cases, a correlation has been established
between the optical properties and the stereochemistry (361).

The four metallocenes mostly used in stereochemical studies are ferrocene (55), cyman-
trene (56) (cyclopentadienyl-Mn-tricarbonyl),
benchrotrene (57) (benzene-Cr-tricarbonyl), and
ruthenocene (58). Formulas (55) to (58) show
their Newman projection. Three isomers of disubstituted ferrocenes, ruthenocenes and benchrotrenes are possible, of which only two, namely

150

the homoannular ferrocenes and ruthenocenes and
o- and m- substituted benchrotrenes are chiral.
Only two isomeric disubstituted cymantrenes are
possible, both of which are chiral (361).

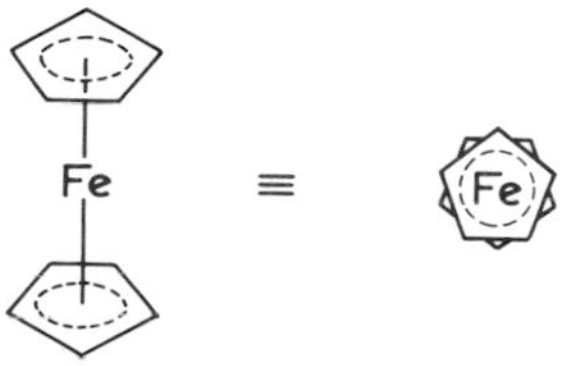

55

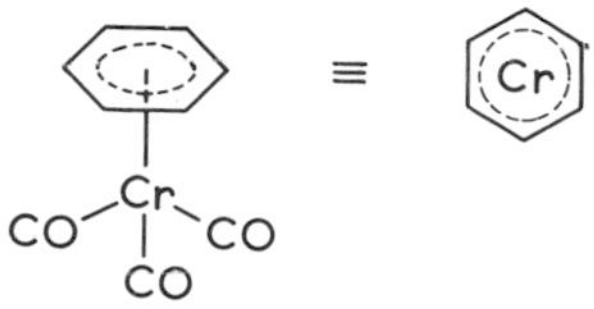

57

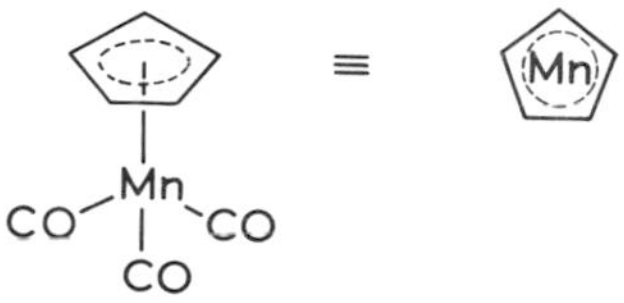

56

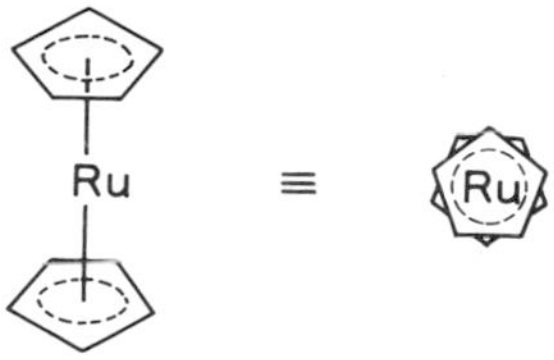

58

        Optically active ferrocenes, ruthenocenes,
cymantrenes and benchrotrenes exhibit a Cotton
effect in the region of 440, 350, 330 and 390 nm,
respectively, corresponding to the long wavelength UV band attributed to a d-d transition.
Analogous cyclic and open chain metallocenes of
identical configuration, exhibit CD curves of
similar shape but of opposite sign, probably indicative of different preferred conformations
(361).
        An empirical rule has been proposed which
establishes a relationship between the configuration, the preferred conformation and the sign of
the rotation at 589 nm. This rotation probably
reflects the sign of the Cotton effect appearing

at high wavelength. When looking at the compound along the molecular axis with the substituent of lower symmetry pointing upwards, if the disturbing chromophoric group (ketone, double bond, etc.) is on the left side, the compound is dextrorotatory. Conversely, if the chromophoric group is located on the right side, a negative rotation is observed (361).

In simple cases, the inherent achiral metallocene chromophore is perturbed by the chiral surrounding and hence becomes active. In cases where no conformational chirality is possible, the magnitude of the Cotton effects is low. However, in ferrocenophanes and biferrocenyls the chromophore itself may be inherently chiral, then rather intense Cotton effects can be observed (361). Recently, other empirical correlations between the Cotton effects and the configuration of ferrocenes have been proposed (362).

References

335. K. Schlögl in Topics in Stereochemistry, N.L. Allinger and E.L. Eliel (edit.), Vol. 1, p. 77, Interscience Publ., New York (1967).

336. J. Fujita and Y. Shimura in Spectroscopy and Structure of Metal Chelate Compounds, K. Nakamoto and P.J. McCarthy (edit.), Chap. 3, p. 156, John Wiley and Sons, Inc., New York (1968).

337. H. Brunner, Angew. Chem. Int. Edit., 10, 249 (1971).

338. B. Bosnich, Acc. Chem. Res., 2, 266 (1969); B. Bosnich and A.T. Phillip, J. Amer. Chem. Soc., 90, 6352 (1968); B. Bosnich and D.W. Watts, J. Amer. Chem. Soc., 90, 6228 (1968); B. Bosnich, Advanced Study Institute on Fundamental Aspects and Recent Developments in ORD and CD, Piza (Italy), September 1971, Abstracts of Papers, p. 37.

339. R. Lazzaroni, P. Salvadori, and P. Pino, Chem. Comm., 1164 (1970).

340. A. Panunzi, A. De.Renzi, and G. Paiaro, J. Amer. Chem. Soc., 92, 3488 (1970).

341. T. Yasui, J. Hidaka, and Y. Shimura, Bull. Chem. Soc. Japan, 39, 2417 (1966); N. Koine, N. Sakota, J. Hidaka, and Y. Shimura, Bull. Chem. Soc. Japan, 43, 1737 (1970).

342. J. Hidaka and Y. Shimura, Bull. Chem. Soc. Japan, 43, 2999 (1970).

343. A.J. McCaffery, S.F. Mason, and B.J. Norman, J. Chem. Soc., 5094 (1965).

344. C.J. Hawkins and E. Larsen, Acta Chem. Scand., 19, 185, 1969 (1965).

345. R.B. Martin, J.M. Tsangaris, and J.W. Chang, J. Amer. Chem. Soc., 90, 821 (1968).

346. F.S. Richardson, J. Chem. Phys., 54, 2453 (1971).

347. A.I. Scott and A.D. Wrixon, Tetrahedron, 27, 2339 (1971).

348. A.J. McCaffery, S.F. Mason, and B.J. Norman, Chem. Comm., 49 (1965).

349. E. Larsen and S.F. Mason, J. Chem. Soc. (A), 313 (1966); R.D. Gillard, Proc. Roy. Soc., 297, A, 134 (1967).

350. S.F. Mason and B.J. Norman, J. Chem. Soc. (A), 307 (1966).

351. K. Ohkawa, J. Hidaka, and Y. Shimura, Bull. Chem. Soc. Japan, 39, 1715 (1966).

352. A.A. Smith and R.A. Haines, J. Amer. Chem. Soc., 91, 6280 (1969); H. Kawaguchi and Sh. Kawaguchi, Bull. Chem. Soc. Japan, 43, 2103 (1970); S. Kaizaki, J. Hidaka, and Y. Shimura, Bull. Chem. Soc. Japan, 43, 1100 (1970); K. Matsumoto, M. Yonezawa, H. Kuroya, H. Kawaguchi, and Sh. Kawaguchi, Bull. Chem. Soc. Japan, 43, 1269 (1970); C.J. Hipp and W.A. Baker, J. Amer. Chem. Soc., 92, 792 (1970); J.H. Worrell, T.E. MacDermott, and D.H. Busch, J. Amer. Chem. Soc., 92, 3317 (1970); H.M. Bössler and R.C. Schulz, Makromol. Chem., 135, 87 (1970); F. Mizukami, H. Ito, J. Fujita, and K. Saito, Bull. Chem. Soc. Japan, 43, 3973 (1970); R. Larsson and B. Norden, Acta Chem. Scand., 24, 2681 (1970); J.E. Sarneski and F.L. Urbach, J. Amer. Chem. Soc., 93, 884 (1971).

353. D. Dodd and M.D. Johnson, Chem. Comm., 571
(1971); R.B. von Dreele and R.C. Fay, J.
Amer. Chem. Soc., 93, 4936 (1971).

354. M. Parris and A.E. Hodges, Canad. J. Chem.,
49, 1133 (1971); K.T. Kan and D.G. Brewer,
Canad. J. Chem., 49, 2161 (1971); H. Ito
and J. Fujita, Bull. Chem. Soc. Japan, 44,
741 (1971); M. Nakai, M. Yoneyama, and M.
Hatano, Bull. Chem. Soc. Japan, 44, 874
(1971); J. Besançon, G. Tainturier, and J.
Tirouflet, Bull. Soc. Chim. France, 1804
(1971); G. Maglio, A. Musco, R. Palumbo,
and A. Sirigu, Chem. Comm., 100 (1971).

355. A. De Renzi, R. Palumbo, and G. Paiaro, J.
Amer. Chem. Soc., 93, 880 (1971).

356. D.L. Caldwell, P.E. Reinbold, and K.H.
Pearson, J. Amer. Chem. Soc., 92, 4554
(1970).

357. R.S. Downing and F.L. Urbach, J. Amer. Chem.
Soc., 92, 5861 (1970).

358. V.Doron and W. Durham, J. Amer. Chem. Soc.,
93, 889 (1971).

359. K.M. Jones and E. Larsen, Acta Chem. Scand.,
19, 1210 (1965); R.C. Fay, A.Y. Girgis, and
U. Klabunde, J. Amer. Chem. Soc., 92, 7056,
7061 (1970); T. Aratani, T. Gonda, and H.
Nozaki, Tetrahedron, 26, 5453 (1970); W.A.
Eaton and W. Lovenberg, J. Amer. Chem. Soc.,
92, 7195 (1970); S. Kaizaki, J. Hidaka, and
Y. Shimura, Bull. Chem. Soc. Japan, 43,
3024 (1970); E. Fujimori and J. Pecci, Biochim. Biophys. Acta, 221, 132 (1970); Y.
Nishida and S. Kida, Bull. Chem. Soc. Japan,
43, 3814 (1970).

360. S.F. Mason, Advanced Study Institute on
Fundamental Aspects and Recent Developments
in ORD and CD, Piza (Italy), September
1971, Abstracts of Papers, pp. 19,39.

361. K. Schlögl, Pure and Appl. Chem., 23, 413
(1970), and references therein.

362. H. Falk and H. Lehner, Tetrahedron, 27,
2279 (1971), and references cited therein.

VII. MAGNETIC OPTICAL ROTATORY DISPERSION AND MAGNETIC CIRCULAR DICHROISM

The intrinsically dissymmetric structure of a chiral molecule induces natural optical activity, i.e. a differential response of the molecule to left and right circularly polarized light. In magneto-optical activity, it is the external magnetic field which provides the proper environment for such a response (385a). Hence, MORD and MCD are not dependent on the presence of an asymmetric center or a chiral structure. If one applies a magnetic field to any optically inactive substance, it becomes optically active. This induced activity gives rise to MORD and MCD curves (15,59). The applications of these techniques in structural chemistry are mainly concerned with studying the nature of the electronic transitions corresponding to a particular absorption. In these measurements one is examining either the activity induced by a powerful magnetic field in symmetrical or racemic substances which are not active or the substantially increased activity induced in compounds which are chiral.

The magnetically induced activity, called Faraday effect (4), is different from natural optical activity. In the Faraday effect, left and right circularly polarized light is passed through a medium, and a magnetic field (H) is applied along the direction of propagation of the beam of light. Since the magnetic field possesses helical symmetry, circular dissymmetry will be produced in the medium, resulting in magnetic-optical rotation α (MORD) and MCD (15,363-367).

MORD and MCD are maximum when the light path is parallel to the applied magnetic field. The sign of the curves depends upon the relative

directions of the light of the magnetic field.
The magnitude of the magneto-optical rotation α
is given by Verdet's equation [9]:

$$[9] \qquad \alpha \; = \; \Lambda \; . \; 1 \; . \; H \; . \; \cos O$$

where H is the magnetic field, 1 is the length
of the light pass parallel to the magnetic field,
Λ is a constant characteristic of the substance
under study and which depends on the wavelength
of the light and the temperature, and O is the
angle between the magnetic field and the direction of the beam of light (363).

Various studies have been devoted to theoretical and experimental aspects of these methods, which require only the addition of a suitable magnet to existing ORD and CD instruments
(15,363-367).

MORD and MCD are related by the Kramers-
Kronig equation [7] (Sec. II-7). Thus, in principle both techniques provide the same information. However, the interpretation of MCD data
is by far easier than MORD curves (364,368).
MCD arises through Zeeman splitting of circularly polarized components, a difference in the
relative populations among the sub-levels in the
ground state, and a difference in the probability of the transitions. The various procedures
currently used to analyze experimental data include gaussian fits, plottings of the ratio of
MCD to absorption versus the logarithmic derivative of the absorption curve shape function, and
the method of moments, the latter being frequent-
ly used (368).

The substances studied so far by MORD and
MCD range from inorganic complex ions (369) to
biological systems of complex conjugated organic
molecules. The Faraday effect, provides useful
information about charge-transfer transitions.
For a simple transition, a MCD curve is generally the sum of three components. One corresponds
to the splitting of the ground state, the excited state or both, in the magnetic field. This
component has an S shape. It is only observed
if the chromophore has some symmetry. The sec-

156

ond component results from variations brought about by the magnetic field in the probability of transition. It has a gaussian shape. The third component depends on the influence of temperature on splitted states by magnetic fields. It has also a gaussian shape and is only present when splitting is possible. These phenomena have been applied to the study of transitions and are useful when they demonstrate the presence of a magnetic moment in the excited states, because MCD then offers an advantage over other spectroscopic techniques which usually do not provide information on excited states (367). This information permits a quantitative verification of various molecular orbital calculations. In addition, some transitions not detected by UV become apparent by MORD and MCD.

Recent examples of applications of MORD and MCD include carbonyl containing organic molecules (364,370,371), various annulene systems (372), aliphatic (373) and simple aromatic compounds (365,374). Moreover, these techniques have been applied to more complex structures, like purine, pyrimidine, and adenosine cyclonucleosides (375), proteins (376), as well as chlorins (377), vitamin B_{12} derivatives (378), chlorophyll (379), manganese porphyrin complexes (380), and iron tetraphenylporphins (381). Recent reports mention the use of MCD to study charge-transfer transitions in several low-spin d^5 hexahalides and low-spin d^6 octahedral hexahalides (382). Finally, MCD has been applied to test an assignment of the ligand-field transitions of CoI_4^{2-} based on a molecular orbital analysis of electron repulsion and spin-orbit coupling (383).

A recent review article on MCD gives the general background of the method and provides a detailed discussion of numerous organic chemical applications, from simple carbonyl containing molecules to annulenes, nucleosides and porphyrins (384). Although this review gives a precise idea of the broad spectrum of substances

which have already been examined by MCD, it is
only quite recently that the first rule has been
proposed for the interpretation of MCD data
(385).
　　　　　Because of the intrinsic difference between MCD and CD, one could anticipate fundamental variations in the nature of information which
can be deduced from these spectra. This does
not mean that MCD does not provide structural
information, but that the structural information
which can be deduced from MCD spectra appears in
a different form and to a different degree. as
compared to CD spectra (385). Indeed, the variety of band shapes and the range of ellipticities
presented in the MCD data of numerous aldehydes
and ketones (371) indicate that MCD is sensitive
to the molecular geometry of carbonyl compounds.
In addition, the MCD curves of such compounds
suggest that structural correlations might be
obscured· by the incursion of vibrational perturbations on an equal level with structural perturbations. Fortunately, a theorem, derived
from group theoretical principles (385a), now permits the development of a simple protocol to relate the structure of a saturated ketone to the
MCD associated with its lowest singlet $n-\pi^*$
transition (385b).
　　　　　The Seamans-Moscowitz theorem states that
the MCD associated with a symmetry forbidden
transition (e.g. the carbonyl $n-\pi^*$ transition)
is of second or higher order in both vibrational
and structural perturbations; furthermore, the
contributions to the magnetic rotational
strengths of perturbations belonging to different irreducible representations are additive
(385a).
　　　　　The consequence of this theorem is that
the signs and relative magnitudes of the partial
magnetic rotational strengths are determined empirically using other molecular spectroscopic
techniques (385b). The assignments of the signs
and relative magnitudes of the partial magnetic
rotational strengths associated with structural
perturbations are as in equations [10]:

$$B(A_2) \begin{cases} > 0 \quad \begin{array}{l}\text{for perturbers dis-} \\ \text{posed to the rear of} \\ \text{the carbonyl carbon}\end{array} \quad [10a] \\[2em] < 0 \quad \begin{array}{l}\text{for perturbers dis-} \\ \text{posed forward of the} \\ \text{carbonyl carbon}\end{array} \quad [10a'] \end{cases}$$

$$B(B_1) \quad > \quad 0 \qquad\qquad\qquad\qquad [10b]$$

$$B(B_2) \quad < \quad 0 \qquad\qquad\qquad\qquad [10c]$$

$$|B(A_2)| \quad > \quad |B(B_1)| \quad \text{or} \quad |B(B_2)| \qquad [10d]$$

An additional rule, which attempts to take account of the troublesome interactions between structural perturbation and vibrational perturbation, may be stated as follows: Any structural perturbation that stabilizes a conformation of a particular symmetry requires substraction of a contribution to a particular component B value.

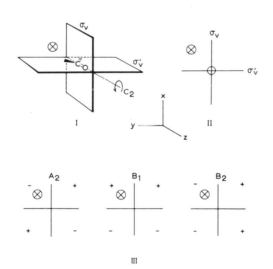

Seamans, Moscowitz, Barth, Bunnenberg, Djerassi,

J.A.C.S., submitted for publication.

Fig. VII-1. Identification and classification of a perturbation due to the extrachromophoric molecular surrounding of the carbonyl group in MCD (385b).

159

The protocol for the identification and classification of a perturbation associated with the extrachromophoric molecular environment of the carbonyl group is illustrated in Fig. VII-1. The symmetry operations of the C_{2v} point group divide the space surrounding the carbonyl chromophore into four sectors, as shown in perspective in I and in planar projection in II (Fig. VII-1). In a perturbation theory treatment, the Hamiltonian operator for the carbonyl chromophore is written as the sum of a zero order Hamiltonian H_0 and the perturbation operator V (equation [11]). In the group theoretical treatment (385a) one has to consider only the symmetry properties of V. This operator may be decomposed into a sum of functions which form bases for the irreducible representations (44) of the point group of the unperturbed system, i.e. the C_{2v} point group in the case of ketones, as shown in equation [11]:

$$[11] \qquad V = V_{A_2} + V_{B_1} + W_{B_2}$$

where the totally symmetric perturbation has been omitted. Reference to the character table for the C_{2v} point group will show that functions belonging to the A_2 representation are symmetric with respect to the C_2 group operation but antisymmetric with respect to reflection in either the σ_v or the σ_v' planes (Fig. VII-1). This behavior is reflected by the pattern of the signed areas in the projection diagram labeled A_2. The sign convention is purely arbitrary and in no way effects the ultimate sign achieved for the magnetic rotational strength. A similar procedure will develop the sign pattern appropriate for structural perturbations of B_1 and B_2 symmetry.

Before applying these symmetry rules to real molecules, one should be aware of the several simplifying assumptions that facilitate the application of these rules. Methyl, ethyl, t-butyl and methylene substituents are taken to be single pseudoatoms. Hence, hydrogen atoms do not appear as perturbers in the diagrams. A further point is that groups lying in the near vicinity of nodal planes, e.g. an α-equatorial methyl substituents, are assumed to contribute less strongly than when well removed from a nodal plane.

A number of applications of these rules has been reported (385b). These symmetry rules are, in principle, applicable to all saturated ketones, although so far the analysis has been limited to such conformationally homogeneous systems as substituted cyclopentanones, decalones, and bicyclic ketones (385).

The MCD rules mentioned above are of much interest for theoreticians and spectroscopists. In addition, since they also give important structural and stereochemical information, one can assume that these rules will have numerous practical applications. The combination of CD and MCD can now provide such a large array of information about the carbonyl group and its vicinity, that one can anticipate that MCD rules will soon become available for other chromophores. This cooperative effort between experimentalists and theoreticians is thus giving a new impulse to ORD and CD on the one hand, and MORD and MCD on the other hand, for the benefit of the scientific community.

References

363. M. Verdet, Compt. rend., 39, 548 (1854); Ann. Chim. Phys., 41, 370 (1954); 43, 37 (1855); 69, 415 (1863); A.D. Buckingham and P.J. Stephens, Ann. Rev. Phys. Chem., 17, 399 (1966).
364. B. Briat, M. Billardon, and J. Badoz, Compt. rend., 256, 3440 (1963); B. Briat, Compt. rend., 258, 2788 (1964); 259, 2408 (1964); 260, 853, 3335 (1965).

365. V.E. Shashoua, J. Amer. Chem. Soc., 82,
5505 (1960); 86, 2109 (1964); Nature, 203
972 (1964); Arch. Biochem. Biophys., 111,
550 (1965).

366. D.A. Schooley, E. Bunnenberg, and C.
Djerassi, Proc. Natl. Acad. Sci. U.S., 53,
579 (1965).

367. B. Briat and C. Djerassi, Nature, 217, 918
(1968).

368. B. Briat, Advanced Study Institute on Fundamental Aspects and Recent Developments
in ORD and CD, Pisa (Italy), September 1971,
Abstracts of Papers, pp. 29,30.

369. A.J. McCaffery, P.J. Stephens, and P.N.
Schatz, Inorg. Chem., 6, 1614 (1967); P.N.
Schatz, A.J. McCaffery, W. Suetaka, G.N.
Henning, A.B. Ritchie, and P.J. Stephens,
J. Chem. Phys., 45, 722 (1966).

370. A.J. McCaffery, G.N. Henning, P.N. Schatz,
A.B. Ritchie, H.P. Perzanowski, O.R. Rodig,
A.W. Norvelle, and P.J. Stephens, Chem.
Comm., 520 (1966); P. Castan, Compt. rend.,
258, 526 (1964).

371. G. Barth, E. Bunnenberg, C. Djerassi, D.L.
Elder, and R. Records, Symp. Faraday Soc.,
3, 49 (1969); G. Barth, E. Bunnenberg, and
C. Djerassi, Chem. Comm., 1246 (1969).

372. B. Briat, D.A. Schooley, R. Records, E.
Bunnenberg, and C. Djerassi, J. Amer. Chem.
Soc., 89, 7062 (1967).

373. H.K. Wipf, J.T. Clerc, and W. Simon, Helv.
Chim. Acta., 51, 1051, 1162 (1968).

374. P.J. Stephens, P.N. Schatz, A.B. Ritchie,
and A.J. McCaffery, J. Chem. Phys., 48,
132 (1968); D.A. Schooley, E. Bunnenberg,
and C. Djerassi, Proc. Natl. Acad. Sci.
U.S., 56, 1377 (1966); B. Briat, D.A.
Schooley, R. Records, E. Bunnenberg, C.
Djerassi, and E. Vogel, J. Amer. Chem.
Soc., 90, 4691 (1968).

375. W. Voelter, R. Records, E. Bunnenberg, and
C. Djerassi, J. Amer. Chem. Soc., 90, 6163
(1968); W. Voelter, G. Barth, R. Records,
E. Bunnenberg, and C. Djerassi, J. Amer.
Chem. Soc., 91, 6165 (1969); D.L. Elder,

E. Bunnenberg, and C. Djerassi, _Tetrahedron Letters_, 727 (1970).

376. G. Barth, R. Records, E. Bunnenberg, C. Djerassi, and W. Voelter, _J. Amer. Chem. Soc._, _93_, 2545 (1971).

377. B. Briat, D.A. Schooley, R. Records, E. Bunnenberg, and C. Djerassi, _J. Amer. Chem. Soc._, _89_, 6170 (1967).

378. B. Briat and C. Djerassi, _Bull. Soc. Chim. France_, 135 (1969).

379. C. Houssier and K. Sauer, _J. Amer. Chem. Soc._, _92_, 779 (1970).

380. L.J. Boucher, _J. Amer. Chem. Soc._, _92_, 2725 (1970).

381. H. Kobayashi, M. Shimizu, and I. Fujita, _Bull. Chem. Soc. Japan_, _43_, 2335 (1970).

382. G.N. Henning, A.J. McCaffery, P.N. Schatz, and P.J. Stephens, _J. Chem. Phys._, _48_, 5656 (1968); A.J. McCaffery, P.N. Schatz, and T.E. Lester, _J. Chem. Phys._, _50_, 379 (1969); G.N. Henning, P.A. Dobosh, A.J. McCaffery, and P.N. Schatz, _J. Amer. Chem. Soc._, _92_, 5377 (1970).

383. B.D. Bird, J.C. Collingwood, P. Day, and R.G. Denning, _Chem. Comm._, 225 (1971).

384. C. Djerassi, E. Bunnenberg, and D.L. Elder, _Pure and Appl. Chem._, _25_, 57 (1971).

385a. L. Seamans and A. Moscowitz, _J. Chem. Phys._, February (1972).

385b. L. Seamans, A. Moscowitz, G. Barth, E. Bunnenberg, and C. Djerassi, _J. Amer. Chem. Soc._, submitted for publication.

APPENDIX

Recently, several communications have appeared dealing with important aspects of ORD and CD methods. In addition, a series of lectures has been published on these topics (386). Some salient results will be mentioned briefly.

Chapter I.-
I-6.-

A theoretical analysis of the n-π* transitions of trans-β-hydrindanone and trans-β-thiohydrindanone has been reported (387). This study provides an interpretation for the fine structure associated with the carbonyl and thiocarbonyl bands and leads to a modified definition of the rotational strength. The C_2 symmetry of the carbonyl and thiocarbonyl is considered with expressions which are derived for non-rigid molecules showing a twofold axis of symmetry. The absorption of trans-β-hydrindanone is divided into a part attributed to transitions polarized along the twofold axis (z axis) and a part due to x,y-polarized vibration-induced transitions. The authors could deduce accurate values for the electric and magnetic transition moments. The vibrational structure of absorption and fluorescence and the latter's low degree of circular polarization are shown to be related to the non-planarity of the carbonyl group in the $^1(n \rightarrow \pi^*)$ state. In the triplet state, a larger non-planarity is probably present. Circular polarization in the fluorescence has been observed when racemic hydrindane was excited with circularly polarized light. In the case of the absorption of trans-

β-thiohydrindanone, an upper limit is found for
the electric transition moment and a lower limit
for the magnetic moment. The luminescence at
-196° and the longest wavelength part of the visible absorption band do not show circular polarization. They are probably singlet-triplet transitions. In addition, there is some evidence
that the thiocarbonyl group is planar in the
triplet and excited singlet state (387).

An application of group-theoretical methods to coupled-oscillator mechanisms of natural
optical activity has appeared (388). A coupled-
oscillator mechanism seems to be responsible for
the observed octant rules of saturated ketones
and chiral olefins. Moreover, it appears that
the one-electron mechanism is of negligible importance in determining these rules (388). Theoretical considerations have appeared on the optical activity of alkyl-substituted cyclopentanones (389).

Chapter II.-
II-4.-

3,17-Dihydroxy-estra-5(10),6-diene (390)
constitutes a notable exception to the helicity
rule for skewed dienes. It displays an intense
negative Cotton effect ($[\theta]_{266}$ -15,940) (391),
although Dreiding molecular models indicate that
the diene chromophore is twisted in the conformation of a right-handed helix.

II-7.-

A discussion of the UV and CD properties
of γ- and δ-substituted ketones emphasizes the
spectroscopic influence of substituents even relatively remote from the carbonyl group (392).
Several recent studies deal with the
chiroptical properties of diones (65,393,394).
In particular, a simple rule, reminiscent of the
carbonyl octant rule, seems to apply to a number
of rigid α-diketones (394).

II-11.-

A detailed report on the absolute configuration of substituted cyano-acetic acids has appeared (395).

II-12.-

The CD data of new chromium (III) (396)
and cobalt (III) (397) complexes of amino acids
have been reported.

II-14.-

The absolute configuration of many secondary alcohols can be assigned from the sign of
the Cotton effect of their o-nitrobenzoate ester
around 330 nm. Alcohols of (R)-configuration
yield esters which present a negative Cotton effect in this region, whilst the same derivative
of alcohols with the (S)-stereochemistry shows a
positive Cotton effect. These optical properties
seem to result from twisting of the normally
planar o-nitrobenzoate chromophore due to steric
interaction with bulky groups of the alkyl component (425).

Dibenzoates of chiral diols display two
CD maxima of similar magnitude but opposite
signs, attributed to a dipole-dipole interaction
between the two ester groups (91,92).

This rule is most useful and the interpretation of the Cotton effects is easy, because
the conformations of benzoate groups are not involved and the magnitude of the Cotton effects
is substantial (177,178). The benzoate chromophore presents three $\pi \to \pi^*$ bands in the UV, _i.e._
at 280 nm the $^1A_{1g} \to {}^1B_{2u}$ (^1L_b) band, at 230 nm
the intramolecular charge-transfer transition,
and at 195 nm the $^1A_{1g} \to {}^1B_{1u}$ (^1L_a) band. In
these transitions, the first and second absorption bands have the transition moments along the
short and long axis of the benzoate chromophore,
respectively. In glycol dibenzoates having interacting chromophores, the intramolecular
charge-transfer band gives rise to two strong

Cotton effects of similar intensity but of opposite signs around 233 (first Cotton effect) and
219 nm (second Cotton effect). The splitting
indicates that both Cotton effects are mainly
due to a dipole-dipole interaction between the
electric transition moments of the intramolecular charge-transfer band of two benzoate chromophores, and that the Cotton effects are separated from each other by a Davydov splitting.
The electric transition moment is approximately
parallel to the alcoholic C-O bond, irrespective
of the rotational conformation around the C-O
bond.
    If chiralities between two benzoate groups
which, to a first approximation, reflect the
chiralities between two electric transition moments, are defined as being positive or negative,
respectively, according to whether the rotation
is in the sense of a right- or left-handed screw
(clockwise or counter-clockwise twist) (Fig. A-1)
then the sign of the first Cotton effect around
233 nm is in agreement with the chirality (398).

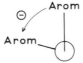

Positive chirality   Negative chirality

K. Nakanishi and N. Harada, unpublished results

Figure A-1. The aromatic chirality method.

The dibenzoate Cotton effects are among the strongest encountered in common molecules. This makes the present rule a convenient method for determining the absolute configurations or chiralities of glycols. Other chromophores usually do not interfere because of the difference in position and intensity of the Cotton effects. However, if necessary, the dibenzoate Cotton effects can be shifted by introducing suitable para-substituents.

The coupling between two benzoate chromophores to give split Cotton effects is not confined to 1,2-glycol systems. Thus, in the cholestane 3β,6β-diol derivative the sign of the Cotton effect is in agreement with prediction. The glycol may also include primary alcohol groups. The nonempirically calculated absolute signs of Cotton effects resulting from interacting benzoate chromophores agree with the chirality of the two aromatic groups. It was expected that the treatment employed in the case of interacting benzoate groups could be extended to other chromophoric groups, such as naphthalene, quinoxaline, as well as an aromatic chromophore already present in the substrate. Moreover, the interaction and hence magnitude of the split Cotton effects are greatly enhanced by employing p-substituted benzoates having intramolecular charge-transfer bands close to that of the substrate chromophore.

The aromatic chirality method has been extended to include various triols and aromatic systems different from benzoates, for which the direction of the long axis transition is known. Hence, this method constitutes a versatile and unequivocal way to assign absolute configurations and conformations to a variety of natural products including terpenoids, antibiotics, sugars and alkaloids (398).

The UV and CD properties of N-monosubstituted and N,N-disubstituted benzamides indicate the n-π* transition of the benzamido chromophore to be responsible for a Cotton effect between two aromatic transitions. A correlation is established between the sign of the Cotton effect and the absolute configuration (399a).

The CD data of a number of optically active butyrophenones have been obtained (399b). From the CD band of the n–π* transition one has deduced that two conformations of the non-planar benzoyl chromophore predominate. This conformational equilibrium is both temperature and solvent-dependent (399b).

II-19.-

ORD has been applied to assign the absolute configuration to a number of piperidine alkaloids (400). This has led to the conclusion that the optical properties of 2-alkyl-1-nitroso-piperidine can be discussed in terms of the sector rule for N-nitrosoamines (212,401,402).

II-21.-

A detailed theoretical and experimental study of the sulfide chromophore has appeared (403). The UV vapor spectrum of dimethyl sulfide shows two main bands in the 200-230 nm region. On going from vapor to solution the 220 nm band loses its structure and is blue shifted. A further blue shift occurs with increasing the solvent polarity. Moreover, the UV in solution reveals a very weak transition on the long wavelength edge of the absorption. In cyclic sulfides, this transition undergoes a red shift as the C-S-C angle decreases on going from larger to smaller rings, and appears around 265 nm in episulfides (three-membered rings).

The UV of methyl sulfoxide and hydrogen sulfide presents a band at 200 nm of the same order of intensity as that in methyl sulfide. Dissymmetric sulfides display Cotton effects in the 200-240 nm region. In cyclic sulfides three Cotton effects appear at about 200, 220 and 240 nm. The intense Cotton effect centered around 235 nm in six-membered ring sulfides is red-shifted to about 265 nm in episulfides, paralleling the UV spectrum.

Briefly, three low energy transitions are observed in cyclic dialkyl sulfides. These three bands are optically active in dissymmetric sul-

fides. The very weak band at about 240 nm is assigned to an electric dipole forbidden, magnetic
dipole allowed $b_1 \rightarrow b_2^*$ transition. The second
band around 220 nm is attributed to an electric
dipole allowed $b_1 \rightarrow a_1^*$ transition. The 200 nm
band of moderate intensity is attributed to an
atomic-like $b_1 \rightarrow 3d$ transition (403).

III.-

An interesting example of intermolecular
charge-transfer occurring with a Δ^4-3-keto-ring
C aromatic steroid has been reported (80c). Solvent effects have been observed in the ORD and
CD curves of N-dithiocarbethoxy-amino acids (404).
A paper appeared on the ORD and CD properties of
adenine-8-cyclonucleosides (405). The phenomenon
of induced optical activity has also been discussed in some detail (406).

A recent paper reports the use of solvent
and temperature effects in ORD and CD for the
study of conformational problems (407a). The CD
data of several tetralins and tetralones have
allowed to assign the conformation to their
cyclic system (407b).

IV.

The chiroptical properties of nucleic
acids and polynucleotides have been reviewed
(408). The relatively small optical activity of
mononucleotides and nucleosides is explained by
the fact that the bases have a π electron system
with planar symmetry and hence are not optically
active. The small optical activity must be
caused by the perturbation of the base by the
dissymmetry of the sugar moiety. The sign and
magnitude of the near UV Cotton effect seems to
depend on the orientation of the base relative
to the sugar. Natural purine nucleosides found
in DNA and RNA β-D-nucleosides give rise to a
negative Cotton effect, whereas the corresponding
β-L or α-D compounds show a positive Cotton effect. An additional factor is the nucleoside
conformation, i.e. the orientation of the sugar

relative to the transition dipole moment of the base. The two orientations known to be sterically possible are <u>anti</u>, in which the purine imidazole ring is <u>directed</u> above the plane of the sugar, and <u>syn</u>, in which the base has rotated by 180° around <u>the</u> C_1-N glycosidic bond. This

interpretation accounts for the negative Cotton effect exhibited by purine derivatives and the positive Cotton effect shown by the pyrimidine analogues. In polynucleotides and nucleic acids, new bands appear which were not detected in mononucleotides. In these natural polymers the base chromophores are in a dissymmetric surrounding due to the helical structure. These various factors are considered from a theoretical viewpoint (408).

V-1.-

Empirical, semi-empirical and theoretical calculations of CD and ORD curves of natural polymers have been discussed (409).

Poly-γ-(1)-menthyl glutamate and poly-β-(1)-menthyl aspartate have been synthesized and the secondary structure of these polymers have been studied in order to investigate the effect of the side chain on the polypeptide structure (410). More recently, the synthesis of poly N-(1)-menthyloxycarbonyl-L-lysine has been reported along with the optical properties showing its secondary structure (411).

An important paper devoted to polypeptides and proteins indicates that their chiroptical data allow to study the fundamental optical properties of the various molecular groups present in such systems, as well as to ascertain the conformation of proteins in solution (412). In addition, these methods allow to investigate changes in molecular structure under a variety of chemical and biological conditions (412). It is also shown that besides the peptide moiety, the molecular groups in proteins, which have significant UV absorption are the aromatic chains of tryptophan, tyrosine, and phenylalanine, as well as the disulfide groups of cystine residue. Small

contributions to the optical activity also result
from the presence of carboxylate and ammonium
groups. The presence of a metal in some proteins
can modify the UV and optical properties of the
molecular groups with which the metal is associated. Generally, the contributions of these
groups to the chiroptical spectra of proteins
are relatively small compared with peptide groups
for two reasons. First, the relative numbers
of such groupings are small. Second, the inherent optical activity of these groups is lower
than that of the peptide groups (412).

The CD curves of aromatic hydrocarbons
and quinolines bound to DNA exhibit a positive
or a negative Cotton effect in the region of absorption of these small molecules bound to DNA
(413). In the denatured DNA-proflavine or RNA-
proflavine complex, a new CD pattern is observed,
which is attributed to a dye-dye interaction.
Induced Cotton effects were also observed for
complexes with a single-stranded DNA, obtained
by dilution denaturation at neutral pH. This
seems to indicate that even the single-stranded
DNA retains some rigidity in which helical structure is maintained by interbase stacking (413).

In contrast to a previous report (315),
recent studies have failed to show that LSD has
any effect on DNA conformation (414). The CD
curves of a number of superhelical DNA have been
obtained. The introduction of negative superhelical turns induces an increase in magnitude
of the positive Cotton effect around 280 nm,
whereas the minimum around 250 nm is hardly affected (415).

Alteration of the DNA ellipticity bands
in presence of a variety of neutral salts and in
dioxane solution have been reported (416). A
careful comparison between UV and CD data of sus-
pension of red blood cell membranes indicates,
in particular, that the molecular ellipticity at
222 nm is not significantly influenced by arti-
facts, and that in the intact membranes, the protein is on the average about 40% in the right-
handed α-helical conformation (417).

V-2.-

ORD and CD of synthetic polymers can provide useful information on the conformational
equilibria of these macromolecules in solution
(418). Neighboring interactions between chromophores present in monomeric units, a common phenomenon in peptides and proteins, is not frequent
in synthetic polymers. However, sometimes the
chromophoric system of the polymer is different
from that of the monomeric unit. Such is the
case of linear poly-acetylenes and poly-iso-
cyanates. In both cases the high intensity CD
bands appear in the UV region where electronic
transitions connected with the existence of par-
tially conjugated monomeric unit chromophores
are expected. This is interpreted as due to a
predominant helical sense of the conjugated main
chain double bonds. Using experimental and theoretical data of poly-α-olefins, so far the only
series of synthetic polymers in which quantitative studies and calculations have been possible,
poly-vinyl-ethers and poly-vinyl-ketones have
been investigated (418). No noticeable interaction between an ethereal or ketonic group present
in a lateral chain has been detected. Usually,
the intensity of the Cotton effect is larger in
polymers than in models. In addition, it increases with increasing stereoregularity. The
same applies to copolymers of α-olefins with
styrene in which a CD of remarkable intensity
has been observed. It corresponds to the lowest
energy π-π* transition of the aromatic chromophore. Its sign is connected with the prevailing helical conformation of the copolymer main
chain.

The most general conclusions have been
reached in the case of vinyl polymers and copolymers in which the existence of one prevailing
ordered helical conformation must be present.
This conformation usually results from a relatively small number of allowed conformations for
each monomeric unit inserted in a vinyl polymer
chain. The small number of allowed conformations
causes a substantial increase of the intensity

of the Cotton effect related to the paraffinic
backbone of the monomeric units, as well as of
the Cotton effects associated with intrinsically
non dissymmetric chromophores present in lateral
chains. The increase of the Cotton effect intensity is related to the prevalence of main chain
conformations with a simple screw pattern, and
thus is dependent on the main chain stereoregularity (418).

References

386. Advanced Study Institute on Fundamental
     Aspects and Recent Developments in ORD and
     CD, Abstracts of Papers, Pisa (Italy),
     September 1971.
387. C.A. Emeis and L.J. Oosterhoff, J. Chem.
     Phys., 54, 4809 (1971).
388. P.J. Stiles, Nature Phys. Sci., 232, 107
     (1971).
389. F.S. Richardson, D.D. Shillady, and J.E.
     Bloor, J. Phys. Chem., 75, 2466 (1971).
390. F. Alvarez and A.N. Watt, J. Org. Chem.,
     in press. Thanks are due to Mr. F. Alva-
     rez for a copy of the manuscript prior to
     publication.
391. P. Crabbé, C. Castelazo, R. Contreras, L.
     Cuéllar, E. Galeazzi, and G. Guzmán, sub-
     mitted for publication.
392. M.T. Hughes and J. Hudec, Chem. Comm., 805
     (1971); G.P. Powell and J. Hudec, Chem.
     Comm., 806 (1971).
393. W. Hug, J. Kuhn, K.J. Seibold, H. Labhart,
     and G. Wagniere, Helv. Chim. Acta, 54, 1451
     (1971).
394. A. Rassat and G. Gagnaire, private communi-
     cation; G. Gagnaire, Ph.D. Thesis, Univer-
     sity of Grenoble, September 1971. Thanks
     are due to Dr. Rassat and Mrs. Gagnaire
     for providing these observations prior to
     publication.
395. J. Knabe and C. Urbahn, Ann. Chem., 750,
     21 (1971).

396. H. Mizuochi, A. Vehara, E. Kyuno, and R. Tsuchiya, Bull. Chem. Soc. Japan, 44, 1555 (1971).

397. K. Okamoto, J. Hidaka, and Y. Shimura, Bull. Chem. Soc. Japan, 44, 1601 (1971).

398. K. Nakanishi, private communication; N. Harada, S. Suzuki, H. Uda, and K. Nakanishi, J. Amer. Chem. Soc., 93, 5577 (1971); K. Nakanishi, M. Endo, U. Näf, and LeRoy F. Johnson, J. Amer. Chem. Soc., 93, 5579 (1971); N. Harada and K. Nakanishi, Acc. Chem. Res., in preparation.

399a. W.C. Krueger, R.A. Johnson, and L.M. Pschigoda, J. Amer. Chem. Soc., 93, 4865 (1971).

399b. O. Korver, Tetrahedron, 27, 4643 (1971).

400. H.C. Beyerman, L. Maat, and J.P. Visser, Rec. Trav. Chim., 86, 80 (1967); H.C. Beyerman, L. Maat, J.P. Visser, J. Cymerman Craig, R.P.K. Chan, and S.K. Roy, Rec. Trav. Chim., 88, 1012 (1969).

401. H.C. Beyerman, S. Van den Bosch, J.H. Breuker, and L. Maat, Rec. Trav. Chim., 90, 755 (1971).

402. G. Snatzke, H. Ripperger, C. Horstmann, and K. Schreiber, Tetrahedron, 22, 3103 (1966).

403. A. Moscowitz, in ref. 386, p. 10.

404. K. Ishikawa, K. Achiwa, and S. Yamada, Chem. Pharm. Bull. Japan, 19, 912 (1971).

405. M. Ikehara, M. Kaneko, Y. Nakahara, S. Yamada, and S. Vesugi, Chem. Pharm. Bull. Japan, 19, 1381 (1971).

406. B. Bosnich, in ref. 386, p. 35.

407a. M. Legrand, in ref. 386, pp. 39,41.

407b. J. Barry, H.B. Kagan, and G. Snatzke, Tetrahedron, 27, 4737 (1971).

408. J. Brahms, in ref. 386, p. 51.

409. I. Tinoco, in ref. 386, p. 13.

410. H. Yamamoto, Y. Kondo, and T. Hayakawa, Biopolymers, 9, 41 (1970); H. Yamamoto and T. Hayakawa, Biopolymers, 10, 309 (1971).

411. H. Yamamoto and T. Hayakawa, Bull. Chem. Soc. Japan, 44, 1990 (1971).

412. E. Blout, in ref. 386, p. 46.

413. M. Kaneko and C. Nagata, <u>Chem. Biol. Inter-actions</u>, <u>3</u>, 459 (1971).
414. A.H. Brady, E.M. Brady, and F.C. Boucek, <u>Nature</u>, <u>232</u>, 189 (1971); E.M. Smit and P. Borst, <u>Nature</u>, <u>232</u>, 191 (1971).
415. M.F. Maestre and J.C. Wang, <u>Biopolym.</u>, <u>10</u>, 1021 (1971).
416. A.J. Adler and G.D. Fasman, <u>J. Phys. Chem.</u>, <u>75</u>, 1516 (1971).
417. M. Glaser and S.J. Singer, <u>Biochem.</u>, <u>10</u>, 1780 (1971).
418. P. Pino, in ref. 386, p. 44.

PROBLEMS

- Which is the sign of the $\pi_x - \pi_x^*$ Cotton effect of _trans_-cyclo-octene? [Answer: see Chem. Comm., 43 (1970)]

- Study the sign of the long-wavelength Cotton effect of the steroidal $\Delta^{5,7}$-dienes with the various possible configurations at C-9 and C-10. [Rec. Trav. Chim., 84, 932 (1965)]

- Which are the signs of the Cotton effects associated with the 20-carbonyl group in 16-substituted 20-keto-pregnanes with the four different configurations at C-16 and C-17? [Tetrahedron, 20, 2455 (1964); ref. 14]

- Discuss the Cotton effect exhibited by the 3-keto chromophore in a 5αH- and a 5βH-B-homo-steroid. [Ann. Chem., 747, 123 (1971)]

- What would be the Cotton effect of 1α-Me and 1β-Me 2-keto-A-nor steroids? [J. Chem. Soc. (C), 2422 (1971)]

- Which will be the sign and intensity of the Cotton effect associated with compounds I to IV?

I, $\Delta^{1,2}$

II, $\Delta^{1,3}$

III, $\Delta^{1,2}$

IV, $\Delta^{1,3}$

[Tetrahedron, <u>27</u>, 2481 (1971)]

- α- and β-rotunol are isomeric sesquiterpenoids of structure I. α-Rotunol presents a positive Cotton effect in the 320 nm region and a negative CD band around 240 nm. β-Rotunol shows an intense negative CD band at <u>ca</u>. 340 nm and an intense positive maximum about 240 nm. Assign the configuration to both isomers.

I

[Tetrahedron, <u>27</u>, 4831 (1971)]

- Discuss the Cotton effect associated with the triterpenes I to IV:

I, 2α

II, 2β

III, 3α

IV, 3β

[Chem. Pharm. Bull. Japan, 19, 753 (1971)]

— Which is the Cotton effect shown by these
   (24S) and (24R) isomeric ketones?

[Tetrahedron Letters, 3237 (1971)]

— Discuss the sign and intensity of the Cotton
   effects associated with the 7-keto-group in
   the various diterpenes of structure I with
   different configurations at C-8 and C-12, and
   double bonds located at C-9(11), C-8', C-12',
   Δ^{13}, etc.

I

[Tetrahedron, <u>27</u>, 2385 (1971)]

- Apply the extension of the octant rule to the n-π* transition of conjugated ketones for the calculation of the conformational energy in (+)-pulegone. [<u>Chem. Comm.</u>, 126 (1971)]

- Assign the conformation to (3S,5R)-<u>cis</u> and (3S,5S)-<u>trans</u>-3,5-dimethylvalerolactones. [ref. 123]

- What conclusion can one draw from the fact that 2-methyl-4'-methoxybutyrophenone exhibits opposite Cotton effect CD curves in ethanol at room temperature and in EPA at -185°? [<u>Tetrahedron</u>, <u>27</u>, 4643 (1971)]

- Apply the extended dibenzoate chirality method using Pr(DPM)$_3$ to 5α-cholestane-2α,3β-diol and its 2β,3β,isomer. [ref. 92]

- Which Cotton effect do you predict for L-α-amino-n-butyric acid? [ref. 138]

- Which sign do you predict for the n-π* Cotton effect of <u>cis</u>-amino-L-proline? [<u>Tetrahedron</u>, <u>27</u>, 4681 (1971)]

- What is the conformation of ring B in $\Delta^{9(11)}$-ring A aromatic steroids and of ring C in Δ^6-ring A aromatic steroids? [ref. 180]

- Apply the aromatic chirality method to assign the absolute configuration to (-)-amurensine I, which presents the following Cotton effects: $\Delta\varepsilon_{215}-8.2$, $\Delta\varepsilon_{230}+8.2$, $\Delta\varepsilon_{242}-3.74$, $\Delta\varepsilon_{278}+2.1$, $\Delta\varepsilon_{290}-5.84$.

I

[Tetrahedron Letters, 3425 (1971); ref. 177]

- Which Cotton effect do you predict for the cyclic ketones Ia and Ib, obtained from veratramine?

Ia, 22βH
b, 22αH

[Tetrahedron, 27, 3387 (1971)]

- Which conformation do you assign to ring B in 3(S)-methyl tetralone, which shows a multiple positive Cotton effect CD curve in the 310-360 nm region? [Tetrahedron, 27, 4737 (1971)]

183

Apply the octant rule to predict the Cotton effect of a 4,4-dimethyl $8\alpha,9\beta$-3-keto steroid, its Δ^7- and its $\Delta^{9(11)}$-analogue. [Tetrahedron Letters, 3463 (1971); ref. 14]

Which is the sign of the Cotton effect of 2α-ethyl-1-nitrosopiperidine and of its 2β-isomer? [Rec. Trav. Chim., 90, 755 (1971)]

TABLES

Table of Rules presently available in ORD-CD

Chromophore	Rule	Figure	References
Allene	Sector	Fig. II-5	85,86
Amino acid	Sector	Fig. II-10	138
Aromatic	Quadrant		149
Aromatic	Sector	Fig. II-12	151
Aromatic	Sector	Fig. II-14	156
Aromatic	Chirality	Fig. A-1	398
Arylazo-group	Sector		216
Azide	Octant	Fig. II-19	209
Azomethine	Chirality		211
Benzoate	Sector	Fig. II-13	91
Carbonyl	Octant	Fig. II-6	22
Carboxyl	Sector	Fig. II-9	121-125
Cobalt (III) complex	Octant		344
Cyclopropyl ketone	Octant		100
Dibenzoate	Chirality		91,178,398
Diene	Helicity	Fig. II-3	43,77
Diene, conjugated ketone, olefin	Allylic axial		65,81
Dithiocarbamate	Quadrant	Fig. II-18	208
Dithiocarbonate	Chirality	Table II-3	72
Epoxyketone	Octant		100
Episulfide	Sector	Fig. II-15	72
α,β-Unsaturated ketone	Octant		108
β,γ-Unsaturated ketone	Octant	Sec. II-10	36,116
Metal complex of pseudo-tetragonal class	Sector (Symmetry)		346
Metal complex with amino acid	Hexadecant		145,343
Metal ion complex	Double-octant		345
Nitrobenzoate	Chirality		425
Nitro-group	Sector	Fig. II-21	215
N-nitroso-group	Sector	Fig. II-20	186,212
Olefin	Octant	Fig. II-1	68,69
Osmate ester	Chirality		75
Peptide	Quadrant	Fig. IV-1	44
Phenylalkylamine, HCl	Quadrant-Sector	Fig. II-17	204
Phosphine oxide	Displacement		235
Platinum (II)-olefin complex	Quadrant		347
Styrene	Chirality		180
Sulfoxide	Displacement		235
Thionocarbonate	Chirality	Table II-4	183
Thiocyanate	Octant	Table II-22	219
Trithiocarbonate	Chirality	Fig. II-3	72

185

Table of Compounds, Functional Groups, and Chromophores

Groups	Cotton Effects (λ nm)	Section	References
Acetate	210	II-11	121,122,126
Acid	210	II-11,12	14,15,121-133
Acylthiourea	340-345	II-21	15,223
Adamantanone	295-300		99
Albumin		V-1	159,282,295,296,302
Alcohol		II-6,14	14,91,217,425
Aldehyde	300	II-7,9,10	14,22,45-48
Alkaloid		II-14,16	12-15,148,165-174, 398
Alkene	180-220	II-3	65-75
Alkylaziridine	260 (290)	II-19	218
Alkyldithiocarbamate	270,330		13,207
Alkylnitrite	320-440	II-16	13-15,188
Alkylsufinyl	210,230	II-21	231
Allene	210-250	II-5	40,79,84-86
Amide	200,215	IV-1	34,44,57,272-279
Amine	200,225	II-16	184
Amino acid	215	II-12,16,17, VI-1,VI;A	12-15,136-146,396, 397,404
Amino alcohol		II-6,II-16	11-15,87,88,136-143
Amino ketone			14,105,148
Aminoindanol	220,270		174
Anhydride	210-220	II-11	14,135
Anilide		II-11	135
Annulene	260,320,390	II-14;VII	164,372
Antibiotic			13,14,161,177,238, 246,247,250,280, 322,398
Aralkylamine	200-300	II-16	42b,148,203,204
Aromatic	200-380	I-6,II-14	14,31,42b,44,148-181
Arsenic complex		VI	353,354,359
Arylazoalkane	330-390	II-19	216
Arylketone	310	II-10,14	14,118,119,419
Arylphosphoryl			419
Aryltetraline	230-245,285		14,148,156
Azide	280-300	II-18	209,210
Aziridine	260 (290)	II-19	218
Azomethine	230-260	II-19	211
Azo protein	330,385,440	V-1	317
Azoxy	215-230,260	II-22	246
Benchrotrene	390	VI	361
Benzamide		A	399a
Benzazocine		II-14	174
Benzene	200-290	II-14	42b,44,156
Benzimidazole	220-280	II-14	174
Benzoate	225-230	II-14	91,176-178,425
Benzquinolizidine	260,280		14,148
Berberine	200-350	II-14	148,167
Bianthryl	200-380	II-14	14,148
Biaryl	200,260,300, 340	I-6,II-14	14,40,116,148,152, 170
Bilirubin		A	14,405
Biopolymer		VI	159,282,295,296,302
Biotin	190-200,240	II-21	228
Biphenylenephosphorus		II-21	236
Butadiene		I-6,II-4	53,55,77-80

186

Olefin	180-220	II-3	65-75,388
Organo-metallic		II-3,IV-3,	15,74,88-90,143-146,
		VI	287,335,336
Osmic ester	450-550	II-3	71,75
Ovalbumine		V-1	159,282,295,296,302
Oxaziran	195,225	II-22	244
Oxime	195-215	II-13	14,65,147
Ozonide		II-22	241
Palladium complex		VI	353,354,359
Paracyclophane			386,421
Peptide	200,220	I-6,IV-1,	30,44,57,272-280,412
		V-1	
Phenyl	200-280	II-14	14,42b,44,148-151
Phenylalanine		V-1;A	42b,159,306,412
Phenylalkylamine	245-270	II-16	203,204
Phenylimide		II-11	135
Phenylosotriazole	225,250-275	II-14	153
Phenylphosphinate	220,270	II-21	236
Phenylthiohydantoin	265,310	II-16,II-21	159,199
Phosphine oxide	220,230-240	II-21	235,236
Phosphine sulfide	260-280	II-21	235,236
Phosphorane		II-3	76
Phthalimide	320	II-16	14,194,195,196
Phytochrome	200-250	V-1	295,296,301,302
Pigment		IV-3;A	13,126,292,293,321,405
Piperidine		A	400,401
Platinum complex		II-3,VI	74,339,340,347,355
Polyacrylic		V-2	15,133,326-328
Polyaldehyde		V-2	15,133,326-328
Polyalkenylether		V-2	15,133,326-328
Polyester		V-2	133,326-328
Polyhydrocarbon		V-2	15,133,326-328
Polyglutamic acid	200,220	V-1	272,273
Polynucleotide		V-1	13,159,295,296,302,316
Poly-olefin		II-22,V-2	14,15,133,252,326-328
Polypeptide		V-1	12-15,275-300
Polysaccharide		V-1	12-15
Polytyrosine		I-6,IV-1,	58,276,306
		V-2	
Porphyrine		IV-3,VII	13,15,161,287-291
Prostaglandin			422
Protein		V-1;A	12-15,282-297,412
Purine		II-14,IV-2,	14,148,154,281,282,
		VII;A	366,408
Pyrazine	220-300	II-14	174
Pyrazole	200-260	II-14	14,148,173
Pyrazoline	330	II-19	216
Pyridine	270	II-14	174
Pyrimidine		IV-2,VII	14,148,154,159,281,282,
			366,408
Pyrrolidine	189-196,215	II-22	249
Pyrromycinone		IV-3	13,161
Quinoline		II-14	148,156,169
Quinone		II-14	14
Quinoxaline	220-250,320	II-14	14,174
Ribonuclease		V-1	159,282,295,296,302,
			306
Ribonucleic acid		IV-2,V-1;A	159,282,295,296,302,
			313,314,413
Ribosome		V-1	159,282,295,296,302
Rhodium complex		VI	353,354,359

190

References

419.   M. Ikehara, M. Kaneko, and Y. Nakahara, Tetrahedron Letters, 4707
       (1968).

420.   A.S. Meyer and E. Hanzmann, Biochem. Biophys. Res. Comm., 41, 891
       (1970); B.A. Pawson, H.C. Cheung, S. Gurbaxani, and G. Saucy,
       J. Amer. Chem. Soc., 92, 336 (1970).

421.   H. Falk, P. Reich-Rohrwig, and K. Schlögl, Tetrahedron, 26, 511
       (1970).

422.   E.G. Daniels, W.C. Krueger, F.P. Kupiecki, J.E. Pike, and W.P.
       Schneider, J. Amer. Chem. Soc., 90, 5894 (1968); O. Korver,
       Rec. Trav. Chim., 88, 1070 (1969); N.H. Andersen, J. Lipid Res.,
       10, 320 (1969); E.J. Corey, Th.K. Schaaf, W. Huber, U. Koelliker,
       N.M. Weinshenker, J. Amer. Chem. Soc., 92, 397 (1970); H. Shio,
       P.W. Ramwell, N.H. Andersen, and E.J. Corey, Experientia, 26,
       355 (1970).

423.   L. Bartlett, N.J. Dastoor, J. Hrbek, W. Klyne, H. Schmid, and G.
       Snatzke, Helv. Chim. Acta, 54, 1238 (1971).

424.   K.D. Philipson, S. Cheng Tsai, and K. Sauer, J. Phys. Chem., 75,
       1440 (1971).

425.   U. Nagai and H. Iga, Tetrahedron, 26, 725 (1970).

AUTHOR INDEX

A

Abe, A., 138 (330), *143*, 187 (330)
Achiwa, K., 73 (197), *103, 171* (404),
  176, 186 (404), 187 (404),
  189 (197)
Adinarayana, D., 84 (222), *105*,
  188 (222), 191 (222)
Adler, A. J., 173 (416), *177*, 187 (416)
Akagi, M., 84 (220), *105*, 191 (220)
Allinger, N. L., 12, *18*, 146 (335),
  148 (335), *152*, 186 (47), 187 (335),
  188 (47, 335), 189 (335), 190 (335)
Altar, W., 11, *17*
Alvarez, F., 166 (390), *175*
Amar, D., 1 (11), *16*, 23 (66), 25 (66), *88*,
  186 (11, 66), 188 (66), 190 (66)
Anand, R. D., 55 (136), 56 (136), *97*,
  186 (136)
Andersen, K. K., 84 (229), *106*, 191 (229)
Andersen, N. H., 190 (422), *192*
Andersen, T. N., 58 (146), *98*, 148 (146),
  186 (146), 187 (146), 189 (146),
  190 (146)
Anderson, G. R., 132 (301), *140*,
  187 (301), 190 (301)
Anderson, H. W., 30 (85), 31 (85), 32,
  90, 185 (85), 186 (85)
Anderson, P., 46 (114), *94*, 188 (114)
Andres, W. W., 64 (161), *99*, 125 (161),
  186 (161), 188 (161), 190 (161),
  191 (161)
Anet, F. A. L., 116 (268), *118*
Angier, R. B., 85 (238), 86 (238), *108*,
  186 (238), 187 (238)
Aota, K., 53 (130), 81 (216), 82 (216),
  96, 105, 185 (216), 186 (130, 216),

187 (216), 188 (130, 216),
  190 (216), 191 (216)
Aquilar-Santos, G., 74 (201), 75 (201),
  103, 187 (201)
Arago, D. F., 1, *15*
Arakawa, H., 64 (162), *100*, 186 (162),
  188 (162)
Aratani, T., 149 (359), *154*,186 (359),
  187 (359), 188 (359), 189 (359),
  190 (359), 191 (359)
Asahi, K., 87 (250), *109*, 186 (250),
  187 (250)
Ashwell, G., 34 (89), *91*, 187 (89),
  190 (89), 191 (89)
Atkins, P. W., 14, 15 (59), *19*, 155 (59),
  187 (59), 188 (59)
Auer, E., 64 (171), *100*, 186 (171),
  188 (171), 191 (171)
Aurnhammer, G., 64 (162), *100*,
  186 (162), 188 (162)
Avigad, G., 58 (141), *97*, 186 (141)
Axelrod, E., 116 (268), *118*
Axelrod, M., 84 (229), *106*, 191 (229)
Ayres, D. C., 64 (163), 69 (163), *100*,
  186 (163), 188 (163)

B

Bach, E., 73 (197), *103*, 189 (197)
Badoz, J., 155 (364), 156 (364), 157
  (364), *161*, 187 (364)
Badr, Z., 80 (211), *104*, 185 (211), 186
  (211)
Baes, M., 60 (155), *99*, 186 (155),
  188 (155)
Baily, E. D., 136 (324), *142*, 187 (324)

193

SUBJECT INDEX

For specific compounds, functional groups, and chromophores, *see also* tables on pp. 185–191